Gender Justice and Development: Local and Global

It is now generally accepted by development theorists and policy-makers that the popular policies of reducing or eliminating social welfare programs over the past several decades have increased inequalities and injustices throughout the world. The authors in this collection focus on the gendered aspects of these inequalities and injustices. They do so by exploring the ethics, values, and principles central to understanding and alleviating real-world problems resulting from a lack of gender justice locally and globally.

Some of the authors offer new theoretical and conceptual frameworks in order to analyse connections between gender norms and inequalities, to devise strategies to empower women and strengthen communities, to challenge mainstream understandings of justice and responsibility, to promote caring and just relationships among people within and across borders, or to shape more adequate accounts of development and global ethics. Other authors apply new theories and concepts in order to explore gender justice in the context of issues such as climate change, land ownership rights in Cameroon, or empowerment strategies in places such as Afghanistan, Bangladesh, Ghana, Columbia, and Indonesia.

This book was originally published as a special issue of *Ethics and Social Welfare*.

Christine M. Koggel is Professor of Philosophy at Carleton University, Ottawa, Canada, and Harvey Wexler Chair in Philosophy, Bryn Mawr College, Pennsylvania, USA. She is the author of *Perspectives on Equality: Constructing a Relational Theory* (1997). Her current research in development ethics explores concepts and issues relevant to a global context.

Cynthia Bisman is Professor Emeritus of Social Work at Bryn Mawr College, Pennsylvania, USA. She has focused her scholarship on the moral core of social work. Her latest book is *Social Work: Value Guided Practice for a Global Society* (2014).

Gender Justice and Development: Local and Global

Volume I

Edited by
Christine M. Koggel and
Cynthia Bisman

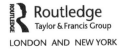
Routledge
Taylor & Francis Group

LONDON AND NEW YORK

First published 2015
by Routledge
2 Park Square, Milton Park, Abingdon, Oxon, OX14 4RN, UK

and by Routledge
711 Third Avenue, New York, NY 10017, USA

Routledge is an imprint of the Taylor & Francis Group, an informa business

British Library Cataloguing in Publication Data
A catalogue record for this book is available from the British Library

ISBN 13: 978-1-138-85255-6

Typeset in Trebuchet MS
by RefineCatch Limited, Bungay, Suffolk

Publisher's Note
The publisher accepts responsibility for any inconsistencies that may have arisen during the conversion of this book from journal articles to book chapters, namely the possible inclusion of journal terminology.

Disclaimer
Every effort has been made to contact copyright holders for their permission to reprint material in this book. The publishers would be grateful to hear from any copyright holder who is not here acknowledged and will undertake to rectify any errors or omissions in future editions of this book.

Contents

For Emily Ann and in memory of Ann

Citation Information

The following chapters were originally published in *Ethics and Social Welfare*, volume 6, issue 3 (September 2012). When citing this material, please use the original page numbering for each article, as follows:

Chapter 1
Gender Justice and Development: Local and Global
Cynthia Bisman and Christine M. Koggel
Ethics and Social Welfare, volume 6, issue 3 (September 2012) pp. 213–215

Chapter 2
Empowerment, Citizenship and Gender Justice: A Contribution to Locally Grounded Theories of Change in Women's Lives
Naila Kabeer
Ethics and Social Welfare, volume 6, issue 3 (September 2012) pp. 216–232

Chapter 3
Unlocking Pathways to Women's Empowerment and Gender Equality: The Good, The Bad, and the Sticky
Patti Petesch
Ethics and Social Welfare, volume 6, issue 3 (September 2012) pp. 233–246

Chapter 4
Empowering Children, Disempowering Women
Jan Newberry
Ethics and Social Welfare, volume 6, issue 3 (September 2012) pp. 247–259

Chapter 5
Implications of Customary Practices on Gender Discrimination in Land Ownership in Cameroon
Lotsmart Fonjong, Irene Fokum Sama-Lang and Lawrence Fon Fombe
Ethics and Social Welfare, volume 6, issue 3 (September 2012) pp. 260–274

Chapter 6

Gender Justice and Rights in Climate Change Adaptation: Opportunities and Pitfalls
Petra Tschakert and Mario Machado
Ethics and Social Welfare, volume 6, issue 3 (September 2012) pp. 275–289

Chapter 7

Integrating Peace, Justice and Development in a Relational Approach to Peacebuilding
Jennifer J. Llewellyn
Ethics and Social Welfare, volume 6, issue 3 (September 2012) pp. 290–302

Chapter 8

Partiality Based on Relational Responsibilities: Another Approach to Global Ethics
Joan C. Tronto
Ethics and Social Welfare, volume 6, issue 3 (September 2012) pp. 303–316

Please direct any queries you may have about the citations to
clsuk.permissions@cengage.com

Notes on Contributors

Cynthia Bisman is Professor Emeritus of the Graduate School of Social Work and Social Research at Bryn Mawr College, USA. Her most recent book, *Social Work: Value-Guided Practice for a Global Society* (2014) provides a framework to promote social justice inclusive of geography and culture. Bisman presents and publishes widely on the moral core of social work, has been the associate editor (North America) for the journal *Ethics and Social Welfare,* and provides a range of editorial functions for journals in the United States and the United Kingdom.

Lawrence Fon Fombe is a Senior Lecturer in Urban Studies and Development Planning at the University of Buea, Cameroon. He is interested in digital cartography as an important tool in managing spatial variations and environmental problems. He received a BA and Doctorat de 3e Cycle in Geography from the University of Yaounde in 1982 and 1989, respectively. He is a holder of a PhD from the University of Buea, Cameroon (2005).

Lotsmart Fonjong holds a PhD in Human Geography from the University of Yaounde 1, Cameroon and an MA in Development Studies from the University of Leeds, UK. He is Associate Professor of Geography. His research interests include natural resource management, women's rights, human rights organizations, and non-governmental organizations.

Naila Kabeer is Professor of Gender and Development at the Gender Institute, London School of Economics and Political Science, UK. Prior to that, she was Professor of Development Studies at the School of Oriental and African Studies (SOAS) at London University, and Professorial Fellow at the Institute of Development Studies.

Christine M. Koggel is Professor of Philosophy at Carleton University, Ottawa, Canada, and Harvey Wexler Chair in Philosophy, Bryn Mawr College, USA. Her book, *Perspectives on Equality: Constructing a Relational Theory* (1997), shapes the foundation for her research interests in the areas of moral theory, practical ethics, social and political theory, and feminism. She is the editor of *Moral Issues in Global Perspective*; co-editor of *Contemporary Moral Issues* and *Care Ethics: New Theories and Applications*; and author of numerous journal articles and chapters in edited collections. Her current research in development ethics explores concepts and issues relevant to a global context.

Jennifer J. Llewellyn is Associate Professor at the Schulich School of Law, Dalhousie University, Canada. She is also Director of the Nova Scotia Restorative Justice Community University Research Alliance (NSRJ-CURA), a collaborative, multi-partner, interdisciplinary research initiative involving university and community partners. She is currently co-directing a project on Restorative Justice, Reconciliation and Peacebuilding with Daniel Philpott at the Kroc Institute for Peace and Conflict Studies.

Mario Machado is a graduate student in the Department of Geography at Pennsylvania State University, USA. His research interests include sustainable development, social justice, and the gender dimensions of climate change.

Jan Newberry is currently Board of Governors Teaching Chair and Chair of the Anthropology Department at the University of Lethbridge in Alberta, Canada. She is the author of *Back Door Java: State Formation and the Domestic in Working Class Java* (2006).

Eric Palmer is Professor of Philosophy at Allegheny College USA. His recent research in development ethics concerns multinational corporate responsibility in developing nations, particularly in cases of resource extraction. He also focuses upon vulnerability and finance, inquiring into for-profit credit schemes directed towards the poor in less developed nations (through microfinance) and in more developed nations (through credit cards and payday lending). He argues that corporate responsibility in each of these areas of business, when viewed through the lens of the capability approach to development, implies specific duties for multinational corporations and for finance capital.

Patti Petesch, a consultant with the World Bank, specializes in qualitative field research on poverty, gender, conflict, and participatory development. She was study coordinator and co-author of the World Bank's *Voices of the Poor* and *Moving Out of Poverty* global research programs, and is currently part of a team that mobilized rapid qualitative assessments in 20 countries as background for the *World Development Report on Gender Equality and Development*. Her newest study, carried out for USAID, is entitled *Women's Empowerment Arising from Violent Conflict and Recovery: Life Stories from Four Middle-income Countries*.

Irene Fokum Sama-Lang received her LLM in International and Commercial Law from the University of Buckingham, UK in 1992 and her PhD in Employment Security from the University of Buea, Cameroon in 2014. She is currently a Lecturer in Land Law, amongst others, at the University of Buea, Cameroon.

Joan C. Tronto is Professor of Political Science at the University of Minnesota, USA. Her ground-breaking book *Moral Boundaries: A Political Argument for an Ethic of Care* challenges the common assumption that physical and emotional nurturing are private, domestic matters unrelated to politics.

Petra Tschakert is an Associate Professor at the Department of Geography and the Earth and Environmental Systems Institute (EESI) at Pennsylvania State University, USA. Her research is on climate change adaptation, social-ecological resilience, and feminist political ecology.

Preface

Christine M. Koggel, Cynthia Bisman and Eric Palmer

This is a two volume publication in the Routledge Special Issues as Books (SPIB) series. The two volumes are connected by the common title of *Gender Justice and Development*. The full title for Volume I is *Gender Justice and Development: Local and Global* and for Volume II it is *Gender Justice and Development: Vulnerability and Empowerment*. Each volume began as a special issue: Volume I, edited by Cynthia Bisman and Christine M. Koggel, was published as Volume 6, Number 3 of *Ethics and Social Welfare* in 2012 and Volume II, edited by Eric Palmer, was published as Volume 9, Number 3 of the *Journal of Global Ethics* in 2013.

The special issues emerged from papers that were given at the Ninth International Development Ethics Association (IDEA) conference at Bryn Mawr College, Pennsylvania, USA in June 2011. Because the College has a long history of educating and empowering women from around the world, Bryn Mawr was selected by IDEA to host its first international conference in the U.S. with the theme, 'Gender Justice and Development: Local and Global.' About 100 participants from around the world presented papers reflecting a diverse range of theoretical, conceptual, empirical, practical, and activist perspectives from work that included philosophy and the humanities, social sciences, social work, development studies, policy studies, policy making, and local and global organizing. In addition to the papers that were selected for the special issues, now re-published in this two volume set, Volume 10, Number 2 of the online journal, *Ethics & Economics/Ethique & Economique* edited by Mario Solis and Jay Drydyk collected several additional papers. This special issue, with papers available in PDF format, can be found at: http://ethique-economique.net/Volume-10-Numero-2.html

The time was right then, as it continues to be now, to explore gender at local, national, and global levels as a key factor in devising policies for addressing inequalities of all kinds and for alleviating poverty and promoting social, economic, and political justice. As the papers in both volumes show, there is no single definition of gender justice and much disagreement among local, national, and international power-holders and those subjected to power about what constitutes gender injustice and how to alleviate or eliminate it. That said, changes envisioned by measures such as improving health care for women and children, recognizing care as work vital to the survival and flourishing of any society, and increasing women's access to education, property, and work outside the home reflect agreement on the key role that women can play when gender is taken seriously in development theory and policy. Among other things, a commitment to implementing these policies can help to remove discrimination on the basis of gender and to alleviate the inequalities and injustices that discriminatory practices and traditions produce. Despite positive changes on a number of fronts, women across the world, in rich as well as poor countries, continue to suffer for lack of power, agency and voice; continue to be vulnerable to ill-health, early morbidity, the effects of climate change, and violence; and continue to endure inequalities of various kinds. To give content to one example, sexual violence is pervasive in war-torn and post-conflict contexts, has been ignored in the armed forces, organized sports, and college campuses in the U.S. and beyond, is evident in Nigeria with the kidnapping and enslaving of young girls, and is seen in the north of England where officials condoned sexual abuse of girls. These cases gaining public attention in 2014 indicate the need to continue placing gender at the forefront of moral, social, and political theory and action. Given these ongoing conditions in the contemporary context, we believe that reaching a wider readership through the re-publication of these two volumes on *Gender Justice and Development* is imperative. We also believe that exposure to and awareness of IDEA's focus on development ethics can help to devise the theory, the policy, and the social activism needed for addressing these conditions.

The International Development Ethics Association (IDEA) is a cross-cultural group of philosophers, social scientists, and practitioners who apply ethical reflection to global development goals and strategies, to North/South relations, and to human and social development in general. Its goals are to promote discussion of the nature of ethically desirable development, of ethical means for achieving development, and of ethical dilemmas arising in the practice of development. IDEA's international conferences aim to share and apply ethical reflection to development goals and strategies and to relations between the 'North' and 'South'; to effect ethically sound development policies, institutions, and practices; and to promote solidarity, mutual support, and interchange among development theorists and practitioners throughout the world.

On this understanding of its goals, it is clear that IDEA views development as needing to identify and address injustices at local, national, and global levels and to understand the intersections of these. Such concerns were promoted in David A. Crocker's seminar on 'Ethics and Third World Development' at the 1984 World Federation of Future Studies meetings at the University of Costa Rica, an event that fostered a Development Ethics Working Group. The organization's more familiar name was introduced at its First International Conference on Ethics and Development, held in 1987 at the same university, and led by Crocker, who held the IDEA Presidency until 2002.[1] The development ethics approach has continued through the history of IDEA, and its concerns are evident in the thematic titles of its later conferences: 'Economic Crisis, Ethics, and Development Alternatives' (Merida, Mexico,1989); 'The Ethics of Ecodevelopment: Culture, the Environment, and Dependency' (Tegucigalpa,

---

1 Consult Lori Keleher, 'International Development Ethics Association (IDEA),' in Deen K. Chatterjee, ed. *Encyclopedia of Global Justice*, Springer, 2011 and 'History of IDEA' at the organization's website, http://developmentethics.org/about-2/.

Honduras, 1992); 'The New Economic Order and Development: Ethical Challenges for the 21st Century' (Santiago, Chile, 1995); 'Globalization, Self-determination, and Justice in Development,' (Madras, India, 1997); 'Poverty, Corruption, and Human Rights: Ethics of Citizenship and Public Service' (Zamorano, Honduras, 2002); 'Accountability, Responsibility and Integrity in Development: The Ethical Challenges in Sub-Saharan Africa and Beyond' (Kampala, Uganda, 2006); 'Ética del desarrollo humano y justicia global' (Ethics of Human Development and Global Justice) (Valencia, Spain, 2009); and 'Gender Justice and Development: Local and Global' (Bryn Mawr, USA, 2011).

In July 2014, IDEA held its tenth international conference, a 30th Anniversary celebration, in its place of birth, San Jose, Costa Rica, with the theme 'Contribuciones desde la ética del desarrollo para un futuro social sostenible' (Development Ethics Contributions for a Socially Sustainable Future). IDEA is committed to ensuring that the best of the papers from its conferences are collected and published, as these volumes show. Similar work is planned as an outcome of the Costa Rica event. We are grateful to Routledge and especially to Kimberley Smith and Emily Ross for recognizing the timeliness and importance of *Gender Justice and Development* and giving these papers new life in this two volume set of the SPIB series.

INTRODUCTION

Gender Justice and Development: Local and Global

Cynthia Bisman and Christine M. Koggel

The past several decades have brought worldwide agendas about rights and justice to the forefront of international policy debates. Throughout the 1990s, UN conferences reflected these areas in opening space for discourse on issues such as women's rights and the environment. While the economic and political crises of the new millennium have slowed the pace of commitments to the pursuit of equality for all, debates about how best to promote equality and justice continue with increasing awareness at local, national and global levels that gender theory and policy is critical in alleviating poverty and promoting economic growth. These features of the global context led to 'Gender Justice and Development: Local and Global' as the theme for the biennial conference of the Ninth International Development Ethics Association (IDEA) hosted 9–11 June 2011 at Bryn Mawr College in Pennsylvania, USA, at which about 100 papers were presented by participants from around the world. This special issue of *Ethics and Social Welfare* collects a small number of the conference papers, many of which were keynote addresses and all of which address the theme of Gender Justice. The authors reflect diverse theoretical, conceptual, empirical and practical perspectives from research areas that include the humanities, social sciences, law and policy.

The theme, 'Gender Justice and Development: Local and Global', is especially timely with recent trends toward diminishment of social welfare and social justice, continuing oppression of women and increasing attention to global issues. In addition to discussions of ethics, values and principles this issue covers practical applications and highlights the at times tragic real-world problems resulting from lack of gender justice locally and globally. The authors in this issue offer new ways of thinking for a discourse to reduce discrimination against women, to strengthen communities toward sustainability and development and to promote caring relationships among people within and across borders even while some nations are reducing supports toward these ends.

The issue opens with three papers that make use of theoretical and conceptual frameworks for understanding gender and analysing injustices. In each case, the authors move between the global and the local to examine possibilities for promoting women's empowerment in specific areas of the world. Naila Kabeer examines the concepts of empowerment, citizenship and gender justice to argue that citizenship, in conferring legal status and making activism possible, can bridge the gulf between institutional change at the level of entrenched gender norms and individual change at the level of empowering particular women. She draws from empirical research of women in Afghanistan and Bangladesh to explore what development organizations can and should do in their efforts to empower women.

The notion of entrenched gender norms is pursued in the second paper by Patti Petesch, who uses the concept of 'stickiness' to delineate bad and good aspects in development projects designed to empower women. The 'stickiness' of gender norms is bad because norms entrench power relations and injustices in ways that are difficult to remove or change. However, the 'stickiness' of innovations is good when they result in development projects that are successful and can take hold. By examining two development projects, one of health in Ghana and the other of microfinance in a conflict-ridden region of Columbia, Petesch shows how attention to the 'twin stickies' can highlight 'local and global pathways to women's empowerment'. The third paper, by Jan Newberry, complicates the analysis of women's empowerment by turning our attention to the ways in which a global context of neo-liberal policies can give meaning to and have a detrimental impact on women in specific contexts. While Indonesia ended its 32-year authoritarian rule in 1997, democracy came with global neo-liberal reform that emphasized the removal of social welfare programs. In Indonesia this now means that the current emphasis on children's empowerment (by the United Nations and NGOs) has childhood care and education programs continue to exploit women's work, as the government did during the period of authoritarian rule, to provide social welfare at the community level.

Lotsmart Fonjong, Irene Sama-Lang and Lawrence Fombe further the gender justice discussion by exploring local land rights in anglophone Cameroon within a global context of women's rights to land. Drawing from empirical data they explore the historical development of customary laws against women's rights to land while considering the societal implications of this custom of gender discrimination with its negative effects of inadequate food, increasing poverty, decreasing choice, impeding sustainable development and perpetuating violence against women. They argue for an inclusive process of broad-based consultation to develop ethically informed gender-based reforms.

In their argument that gender justice must go beyond a rights perspective toward one of transformative change, Petra Tschakert and Mario Machado advocate use of a human security lens to address the power imbalances that enable inequality around gender, as well as of class and other differences. To alter the climate change dialogue, emphasis on caring and connectedness is necessary in encouraging wider participation, thereby increasing the overall potential of individuals, communities and societies. Shifting from studies of vulnerability to assessments of inequality can better connect people in their shared experiences, impede the perpetuation of injustices and fill a critical need in the work toward climate justice.

The final two papers focus on theory, and specifically on relational theory and its challenge to mainstream liberal accounts of justice and responsibility. Jennifer Llewellyn develops a feminist relational theory of justice—what she also refers to as restorative justice—to argue that in its focus on relationships and the goal of building relationships of equal respect, concern and dignity, restorative justice highlights the importance of addressing peace, justice and development as integrated and interconnected aspects of what it means to address injustices and build lasting peace. Restorative justice, she argues, is in stark contrast to retributive justice and its focus on individualized punishment of wrongdoers as the way to address past injustices. In the final paper, Joan Tronto develops an account of relational responsibilities, one that departs from standard accounts of partiality to sketch a partialist and rich account of the complex nature of relationships and to defend a robust account of our responsibilities to others (Koggel & Orme 2010, 2011). The result is an argument for a global ethics that explains the responsibilities of people in rich countries to those in poor countries in relational terms. An account of partial connections of relational responsibility asks us to do the hard work of assessing values and relationships in order to determine our concrete responsibilities to others in a global context.

References

International Development Ethics Association (IDEA) Available at: <http://developmentethics.org/> (accessed 25 May 2012).
Koggel, C. & Orme, J. (2010) 'Care Ethics: New Theories and Applications', *Ethics and Social Welfare*, Vol. 4, no. 2, pp. 188–200.
Koggel, C. & Orme, J. (2011) 'Care Ethics: New Theories and Applications: Part II', *Ethics and Social Welfare*, Vol. 5, no. 2, pp. 107–9.

Empowerment, Citizenship and Gender Justice: A Contribution to Locally Grounded Theories of Change in Women's Lives

Naila Kabeer

Struggles for gender justice by women's movements have sought to give legal recognition to gender equality at both national and international levels. However, such society-wide goals may have little resonance in the lives of individual men and women in contexts where a culture of individual rights is weak or missing and the stress is on the moral economy of kinship and community. While empowerment captures the myriad ways in which intended and unintended changes can enhance the ability of individual women to exercise greater control over their own lives, it does not necessarily lead to their engagement in collective struggles for gender justice. This paper argues that ideas about citizenship, as both legal status and potential for action, can help bridge this gulf between institutional and individual change. It draws on empirical research from Afghanistan and Bangladesh to explore the extent to which efforts to empower women by development organisations have also encompassed discourses of citizenship which allow them to articulate, and act on, their vision for a just society.

Introduction

This paper is concerned with the relationship between empowerment, citizenship and gender justice. I see these as signposting distinct but interrelated pathways of social change in women's lives which can, but do not necessarily, overlap. I understand women's empowerment to have an irreducibly subjective component. Whatever else, it must entail changes in women's consciousness, in the way they perceive themselves and their relationships with others. It thus begins with individual change. Gender justice concerns the institutional arrangements that govern society including, but not only, its legal system—and the extent to which these promote the fair treatment of men and women. Struggles around gender justice are then struggles around notions of fairness at the institutional level. I will be arguing that ideas about citizenship offer an important bridge between these two processes of change because they help to mediate the translation of individual notions of selfhood into socially recognised identities.

In formal terms, gender justice refers to international norms and conventions relating to women's rights as well as various forms of national legislation seeking to promote gender equality. While there are various factors behind this emerging architecture of rights, a major driving force has undoubtedly been the efforts of feminist activists who see the formal recognition of women's rights as a critical pathway to substantive gender justice. However, legal gender equality has not necessarily translated into gender justice where it matters most: in the everyday life of millions of men and women, most of whom have not taken any part in these efforts and many of whom may not even know that they exist.

At the same time, various intended and unintended forces have been acting on some of the long-standing patriarchal constraints that limit women's agency in everyday life: these include rising levels of education, increasing rates of labour force participation as well as a variety of development interventions, many targeted explicitly at women such as microcredit, cash transfers and reproductive health. Yet, as various studies have shown, women's individual empowerment has not translated everywhere into greater awareness of their rights or greater willingness to act on them.

This paper explores how interactions between women's empowerment, citizenship and struggles for gender justice play out in societies in which ideas about gender equality and women's rights have very shallow roots because individuality itself as a way of life has little or no place. I begin in the next section by discussing efforts to formulate these concepts in ways that take account of the challenges posed by such contexts, starting with my own effort to conceptualise women's empowerment.

Empowerment, Citizenship and Gender Justice: Conceptual Approaches

My definition of empowerment takes choice as its central concept (Kabeer 1999). I defined empowerment as the processes of change through which those who have been denied the capacity to exercise choice gain this capacity. However, I qualified the notion of choice in a number of ways to make it relevant to the analysis of empowerment.

My first qualification related to the conditions in which women make their choices. For choice to be meaningful there have to be alternatives, the possibility of having chosen otherwise. My concern here was with women's apparent compliance with, or at least failure to protest against, norms and values which assigned them an inferior status to men in their society. Such compliance can be variously interpreted. It may reflect an unquestioning acceptance of these norms and values, the belief that they represent a satisfactory, even valued, way of organising social relationships. It may reflect the material costs associated with protest. Where women are economically dependent on those with power and authority over them, attempts to question the status quo can undermine their primary source of survival and security in their society. Or there may be social costs. If there are strong pressures within society to conform to given norms and values, transgression risks harassment or ostracism.

There is also the question of perceived alternatives. To what extent is it possible for women to *conceive* of having chosen or acted differently? In societies where gender inequalities of personhood are so deeply embedded in the family and kinship relations, so intimately bound up with constructions of the self as gendered subjects, that to question them would be to question the meaning of one's existence, there is little scope for imagining other ways of organising social relations. This touches on Bourdieu's idea of *doxa*, aspects of traditions and norms that are so taken for granted that they take on a naturalised and unquestioned quality.

Two other qualifications related to the consequences of choice. The first concerned the distinction between trivial and significant choices, between the choices that we make on a mundane basis every day of our lives and the more strategic life choices that have profound consequences for the quality and direction of the lives we are able to lead.

The second related to the consequences of choice for the broader structures of inequality that prevail within a society. To what extent do the choices in question undermine, and even transform, these structures, and to what extent do they merely reproduce them? Choices which embody the fundamental inequalities of society, which systematically devalue the self or undermine the capacity for choice of others, are not compatible with most feminist under-standings of empowerment, however active the agency underlying these choices may appear.

Let me now turn to O'Neill's work (1990) for a conceptualisation of gender justice that attempts to take account of the kinds of patriarchal constraints that I am talking about. O'Neill seeks to steer a course between the idealised and relativist approaches which have dominated recent debates on this topic. Idealised approaches, exemplified by much of liberal theory, claim universalism by abstracting from the particularities of persons, such as gender or ethnicity, in favour of the abstract individual as bearer of rights and responsibilities. The problem with this conceptualisation of the individual is that it idealises a free-floating agency that is more easily exercised by men than women because it assumes away the relations of dependence and interdependence which are central to the lives available to most women in the real world.

Relativised approaches, exemplified by much of communitarian theory, explicitly acknowledge differences between people and seek to ground ideas about justice in the discourse and traditions of actual communities. The objection here is that most communities relegate varying portions of women's lives to the domestic sphere. Not only do such approaches fail to take account of women's productive capacities and the practicalities of earning a living that many face but they also endorse the exclusion of women from precisely that 'public sphere' where questions of justice are generally addressed (O'Neill 1990, p. 440).

O'Neill believes that a more adequate account of justice requires abstract principles that are genuinely universal, that steer a course between abstractions that smuggle in idealised accounts of the human agent and context-sensitivity that ends up valorising culturally specific ideals about social relationships. The challenge is to articulate principles of justice that can adjudicate between the inevitably diverging views about desired or acceptable institutional arrangements that prevail in most societies. Justice requires that the basic principles for organising institutional arrangements in the face of such divergence must be ones that could be adopted by any plurality of these diverse actors. This would rule out deception, coercion or violence as the basis for organising social life since anything which promotes the agency of some groups at the expense of others cannot be universally acted on. The institutional arrangements that are adopted by all members of such pluralities on the basis of these principles then become the background conditions for their actions.

To illustrate the applicability of this approach to justice to concrete situations, O'Neill considers the situation of poor women in poor communities. How do we judge whether existing social arrangements that isolate or exclude women or ensure their life-long vulnerability violate principles of justice? This is not a question about the kinds of arrangements that hypothesised rational and mutually independent individuals *would* consent to, the idealised approach, nor is it a question about the kinds of arrangements that people in potentially oppressive situations *do* consent to, the relativist approach. Instead, it is a question about the kinds of arrangements a plurality of interacting agents with finite capacities *could* consent to.

O'Neill suggests that one way to capture what is at issue is to ask: to what extent are the different aspects of any arrangements that structure the lives of oppressed groups ones that '*could have been refused or renegotiated by those they actually constrain*' (p. 455; author's emphasis)? Institutions can only be regarded as just if they allow those who are affected by them the ability to refuse or renegotiate different aspects of the tasks and roles assigned to them. However, O'Neill recognises that the capacity for dissent is not evenly distributed in an unjust society. Existing institutional arrangements frequently undermine women's agency by making disproportionate demands on them to meet the needs and defer to the wishes of others and by limiting their capacity to think and act outside given norms and values. We consequently cannot take their failure to protest against existing institutional arrangements as evidence that these arrangements are just. There is therefore a processual aspect to justice: it requires building the capacity of subordinate groups to play an equal part in shaping the institutional arrangements that govern their lives, including their capacity for dissent.

Ideas about agency—the capacity for choice, consent, renegotiation as well as dissent—are thus central to the conceptualisations of empowerment and gender justice that inform this paper. But while empowerment takes the consciousness and capabilities of individual women as its starting point, gender justice is concerned with the quality of the institutional arrangements that govern social relationships. I would like to suggest that ideas about citizenship can provide an important conceptual bridge between individual and institutional change.

There are, of course, many different ways of conceptualising citizenship, not all of them equally compatible with the kinds of agency that we are talking about here. For instance, liberal conceptualisations of citizenship based on the equality of the rights of individuals as recognised by the state and protected by law suffer from the limitations that O'Neill discusses. They privilege individual rights but take no account of how particularities of identity and social position might differentiate the ability to realise rights. Communitarian understandings focus on the shared norms and values which underpin the mutual responsibilities of the members of a community in pursuit of the collective good. But they also lend themselves to the defence of long-standing hierarchies within communities which give little or no voice to subordinate groups in defining what constitutes the collective good.

My aim here is not to adjudicate between different approaches but to draw on the conceptual resources they offer in order to propose the idea of citizenship in different contexts as *work in progress*, an ongoing project that evolves through struggles and contestations between different groups within a society. I want to explore these struggles and contestations through what Lister (1997) describes as the dialectical relationship between citizenship as *status* and citizenship as *practice*. Drawing on her distinction, I will be using the concept of 'status' to refer to how the existing constitutional/legal arrangements in a society define the rights and responsibilities of citizenship, including its gender dimensions, while I will use 'practice' to refer to the different ways in which members of a society seek to act on—and challenge—these collective definitions. While the status of citizenship spells out the possibilities and constraints that individuals and groups experience as members of a particular society, the practice of citizenship places the question of human agency, including the capacity to accept, to conform, to question or to dissent, at the heart of contesting views about citizenship.

Contestations around Gender Equality and Women's Rights

Let me turn next to some examples of communitarian perspectives on women's rights and gender justice to illustrate what I believe to be their limitations. My first example comes from Menon (2000) who uses her research on upper caste

Brahmin women in urban Orissa to reject the universalist assumptions underlying feminist demands for 'equality, individual rights and personal choice' (p. 77). She suggests that the failure of (Westernised) Indian feminists to energise Hindu women to fight gender injustices, or even to protest against them, reflects the fact that such demands are rooted in 'an ideology of individualism' which has no traction for women she researched.

According to her, the women in her study consider themselves complementary, not subordinate, to men. They gain their deepest sense of who they are through their ability to fulfil the destiny of marriage and motherhood laid out for women in Oriya Hindu culture. As a result, many of the practices that feminists have identified as manifestations of patriarchal control are actively embraced by these women in their efforts to live up to twin cultural ideals of self-denial and service to others which define their roles as mothers and wives.

Menon illustrates this claim with a discussion of the practice of female seclusion among the Hindu upper castes. She points out that Hindus believe the human body to be relatively unbounded and permeable and hence subject to continuous change and reconstitution through contacts with others. Upper caste Hindus therefore observe various daily practices and rituals through which they seek to 'refine and regulate' themselves. Since women's bodies are considered more permeable than those of men—because they menstruate and reproduce— they are more concerned than men with regulating exchanges with others who could threaten this process of refinement (p. 81).

Consequently, the women in Menon's study choose to remain within the family compound, restricting their social interactions to family and kin and meticulously observing the prescribed daily practices of ritual purification:

> Strange as it may sound to modern ears, Oriya Hindu women do not desire to move and interact with people indiscriminately. They value, positively, their lack of geographical mobility and their limited interaction with the outside world, interpreting these features as signs of their superiority over others, of their independence of the outside world...To shun contact, to maintain exclusivity, confers a mark of distinction on the person who shuns. (p. 88)

Barakat and Wardell (2002) also question the universality of individual rights, this time in the context of Afghanistan. They argue that those unfamiliar with Afghan culture tend to take women's absence from the public domain as evidence of their subordinate status but overlook the private domain of family and kinship where Afghan women find their primary source of security and status and exercise most influence. To look at Afghan society through a Western feminist prism fails to take account of the concepts and obligations that underpin women's power within the family and the role of patriarchy in providing them with shelter and security. The revered status of women inscribed in the local culture is upheld by Qu'ranic teachings and by Afghan women themselves. Regardless of differences of ethnicity, location and class, women's roles as wives and mothers are central to their identity: 'No matter how vital a woman's economic contribution to her family's well-being, this remains of secondary importance to her position as wife and mother' (p. 918).

Both papers thus reject individualised notions of personhood. Both strongly emphasise women's association with the domestic domain as well as the satisfaction and status they receive from it. Both, however, are flawed by their treatment of culture and community as seamless, timeless and internally coherent. Neither allows for the possibility that any of the women within these cultures might feel oppressed by the predetermined nature of their roles in society and seek to protest against, however silently, their lack of choice about the lives they lead.

A somewhat different perspective on communitarian constructions of identity and personhood is to be found in Joseph's analysis of kinship and family relations in Lebanon (1994, 1997). She notes that the rights of citizenship embodied in the Lebanese constitution played very little role in the lives of men and women in the working-class neighbourhoods of Beirut that she studied. Instead, both men and women experienced their rights as emerging from sets of relationships within which they were embedded as concrete persons rather than as abstract individuals. These 'relational rights'—she borrows the term from Nedelsky (1993)—had a strong gender dimension. The relationships in question constructed gender identities through socialisation processes that stressed *interdependence* rather than *separation* as the basis of gender roles and responsibilities for *both* men and women. Consequently, they promoted connective notions of selfhood for both, 'one that [saw] itself embedded in others and foster[ed] relationality as a central charter of selfhood' (Joseph 1997, p. 86). Notions of selfhood were thus constituted by claims and obligations generated through, and embedded within, the social relationships of kinship, family and community. Nor was this relational under-standing of claims and obligations confined to the domestic domain. Rather, they pervaded all domains of social interaction, rendering irrelevant the idea of an impersonal public sphere in which individual citizens enter as bearers of rights, equal in the eyes of the law.

But while Joseph also questions the relevance of liberal notions of individual rights in the context of her study, and emphasises the 'relational' basis on which rights operate, she is clear that these relationships are rooted in, and reflective of, a highly patriarchal organisation of family, kinship and community. This clearly has problematic consequences for women—as individuals and as citizens. It means that in both the private and public spheres of life they must defer to patriarchal authority figures who mediate their access to valued private and public resources. We might also add that the near-dominance of kinship relations, idiom and morality in all spheres of life means that the only discourse available for the expression of dissent from the patriarchal norms and values of kinship is the discourse of kinship itself.

Despite variations in their recognition of power as an aspect of gender relations, all three papers underscore the conundrum that motivates this paper. How do struggles for women's empowerment and gender justice take place within communities in which the patriarchal relationships of family and kinship not only define gender roles and identities within the domestic domain but also provide the dominant model of relationships in all spheres of society? It is not simply, as Kandiyoti (1988) suggests, that women in such contexts may actively resist individual rights if these are seen to undermine the traditional protections that accompany their dependent status within the family. It may also be the case that they simply do not view these social arrangements as *unjust*. As Basu argues:

> The internalisation of norms over generations means that subjective perceptions about inequality and subordination need have no connection with an outsider's views on these matters. And nor is it clear that one view is more real than the other. (1996, p. 56)

Such views pose a major challenge for feminist concerns with women's empowerment and gender justice as conceptualised in this paper. Recognition of injustice must clearly precede struggles for justice, but if injustices are ingrained in the social relationships that construct women's sense of self and security within their communities then they are likely to be ingrained in women's gendered subjectivities. Is it possible for women to recognise and deal with the injustices embedded in the social relationships that define their identities and give meaning to their lives without at the same time negating or undermining these relationships?

One way out of this conundrum is provided by Benhabib (1992). She notes that a central insight of Habermas's theory of justice is precisely the importance of social relationships in the construction of identity and consciousness: 'The "I" becomes an "I" only among a "we" in a community of speech and action. Individuation does not precede association; rather it is the kinds of associations we inhabit that define the kind of individuals we become' (p. 71). However, she goes on to argue, acknowledging the value and significance of social relationships in people's lives is very different from the uncritical and socially conformist acceptance of their ascribed 'station and duties in life' that features in some of the communitarian literature.

However socially embedded women—and men—may be in the ascribed relationships of family, kin and community, it is in principle possible for them to attain a reflexive distance from these relationships, to become simultaneously observers of, and participants in, their own society. If it is through the 'given' relationships of family and kinship that women gain their sense of identity and personhood, then it is through participation in other 'chosen' forms of associational life that they may be able to acquire a reflexive vantage point from which to observe and evaluate these relationships.

What is appealing about this conceptualisation is that it implies a sense of self and identity that is not predetermined and fixed by cultural norms but shifting and fluid, in constant process of construction and reconstruction through the social interactions of everyday life. It is, of course, possible that the expansion of associational possibilities leads to the reinforcement of old orthodoxies or the rise of new ones, to the substitution of dependency within the home for exploitation at work. But equally, it is possible that it will strengthen women's capacity to recognise and articulate what they consider to be unjust about their lives, to decide what action to take and through their actions come to formulate their vision of gender justice.

This offers a different route to 'relational rights' to the communitarian version that Joseph describes in the context of Lebanon. If, as Nedelsky has suggested, the rights recognised by a society reflect collective choices about the kinds of social relationships it seeks to foster, then the inclusion of previously marginalised groups in the processes of collective decision making may serve to recast the vision of community and redefine the collective good along very different lines to that embodied in the prevailing status quo.

In the remainder of this paper I will be drawing on the findings from two of my recent research projects to illuminate some of the ways in which expanding the sphere of women's social interactions can bring about positive changes in their lives, even in apparently oppressive circumstances, and to evaluate these changes through the conceptual framework outlined in this paper. The women interviewed in both contexts spoke of familial relationships in terms of a patriarchal contract rooted in religious beliefs and cultural traditions. Men were the family breadwinners and guardians of its honour while women were responsible for bearing children, caring for the family, looking after the household and upholding the family honour through their virtuous behaviour.

Development NGOs were the key form of 'chosen' associations on which the research focused and both projects used women's accounts of their life histories to assess their experiences. The first project was based on interviews carried out in Kabul in 2009 with 12 Afghan women and their families (Kabeer *et al.* 2011). They were all from the minority Hazara community and came from poor and lower middle-income households. The women were associated with two development NGOs which provided microcredit to women. Such NGOs are relatively new in Afghanistan and both had started operations in Afghanistan within the previous five or six years.

The second project was based on interviews carried out in 2006 with 31 women drawn from low-income households in rural Bangladesh (Kabeer 2011). These women were associated with four development NGOs, all committed to a lesser or greater extent to women's empowerment, with one providing microcredit and the other three using a savings-based approach. NGOs have had a long history in Bangladesh and many of these women had been members for 10–15 years.

Women's Narratives of Change in Urban Afghanistan

The Hazara women in our study were very explicit in articulating their views about the contractual basis of family life. They prioritised their duties to the family and looked to men to prioritise theirs. They remained within the vicinity of their own homes and were generally accompanied, sometimes by children, if they had to go further. The virtuous woman, in their view, complied with these norms and accepted her husband's right to beat her if she failed to do so. In return, she could expect to be provided for, protected from harm and represented in the public domain.

However, the lived reality that the women described rarely matched up to this idealised version. High levels of male unemployment in a war-disrupted economy made it difficult for men to live up to their obligations as primary breadwinners, leading them to vent their frustrations on their wives and children. Almost every woman in our sample had experienced violence, usually at the hands of husbands. Their struggles to deal with the marked disjuncture between the normative model of the patriarchal contract and its concrete manifestations in their daily lives spelt out some of the forces of continuity and change that have characterised Afghan society in recent decades.

There were clearly a variety of pressures on women to put up with their situation, regardless of how they felt: the weight of tradition, their own adherence to its values, the authority exercised by dominant family members, pressures imposed by the wider community combined with their fear of losing their children in case of divorce, of being sent back in shame to their parents' home were all powerful forces in reinforcing the status quo.

Men too found the burden of breadwinning responsibility difficult to deal with. The stresses they faced could be glimpsed in their own descriptions of their struggles to earn a living and in women's frequent descriptions of husbands as 'bad tempered', 'moody', 'anxious' and 'tense', often combined with an understanding of their frustrations: 'poor him, he has to work from morning till night'; 'poor him, he lost his job'.

However, husbands' behaviours were not only explained as individual aberrations but also as manifestations of a more generalised pattern of injustice that gave men a monopoly on rights and privileges. These women did not subscribe to some monolithic notion of Afghan values. They distanced themselves from the values of the Taliban, for instance, resenting the impositions that it had placed on men and women, particularly from the minority Hazara community. Nor were their expressions of dissatisfaction confined to life under the Taliban. While they did not reject the norms and values of their own communities, they felt a keen sense of injustice that recurring violations of their contractual obligations by men went unnoticed, unpunished and even condoned.

This ability to take a critical stance towards their own society was in part a product of some of the changes that they had lived through in recent years. For some, time spent as refugees in Iran had provided an alternative vantage point, an 'observer status', from which to evaluate their own society. That it was also an Islamic state meant the comparison carried greater weight. One woman contrasted the treatment of women in Afghanistan to what she had observed in Iran: 'Iran is really good from this point of view. You can't put pressure on women. Here they look on women as a slave.'

For others, the experience of life under different kinds of regimes had helped to crystallise the importance of some of the freedoms that they had previously enjoyed and that had been suspended for a period of time, including some degree of mobility in the public domain, the ability to watch TV, to vote, to work, to visit their shrines and to send their daughters to school.

Along with the restoration of these freedoms by the present regime, there had been other changes. Key among these was the emergence of a new legalistic discourse around gender equality and women's rights, actively promoted by the international community and by their own aid-dependent government. Both women and men learnt about this evolving discourse from their televisions, their forays into the public domain and their interactions with each other. TV, in particular, had become an important vehicle for conveying competing discourses about women's place in Afghan society: the discourses of religious leaders combined with educational programmes about women's rights and Indian soap operas which opened a window into women's lives in countries not far away from their own.

There were conflicting views among the women in our sample with regard to this emerging discourse of rights. Some regarded the idea of equality with men as a direct contravention of their fundamental beliefs: how was it possible for women to go out of the house without their husband's permission? Others questioned men's monopoly of power within the 'moral economy' of the community and the absence of any mechanism to restrain their misuse of their privileged position. They welcomed the emergence of alternative forms of jurisdiction, exemplified by constitutional and legal recognition of gender equality, as a means of holding men accountable for their actions and offering some redress to the inequalities of the patriarchal contract.

Given the turbulence of recent decades, it is not surprising that the changes associated with women's access to microfinance appeared relatively minor. In addition, the efforts made by the microfinance organisations to gain acceptance within the community, the absence of any forms of support apart from the provision of credit, and the failure to nurture stronger associational bonds among their members all curtailed their transformative potential.

Nevertheless, where households had made successful use of these loans not only did they experience improvements in their standard of living but it was also possible to discern some of the less tangible gains associated with ideas about individual empowerment outlined above. As the main conduits through which this new resource entered their households, there were reports of greater voice and influence in their households as well as greater respect within their local community. Association with microfinance organisations also served to widen women's sphere of social interactions: through meeting with other women from their loan group, through visits to the NGO office or, in the case of the woman who had set up her own businesses, through daily interactions with their customers: 'The hairdressers is the best place to have a chance to talk to other women like myself. Everybody has their problems especially because Afghan men are so cruel.'

However, there was little evidence that access to microfinance had strengthened women's voice in the wider community or their capacity to act collectively against the injustices they spoke of so eloquently. This may change with the next generation. It was striking how many women in our small sample were using the meagre resources at their disposal to educate their daughters in the hope of carving out what we termed an 'inter-generational pathway of empowerment' (Kabeer *et al.* 2011).

Women's Narratives of Change in Rural Bangladesh

Bangladesh has a long history of development NGOs, dating back to the aftermath of independence in 1971. While many began with a very radical analysis of the structural roots of poverty and focused on mobilising landless men and women, they have become gradually de-politicised over time, taking on an increasing service provision role, with many specialising in microfinance. The focus of our research was on four rural organisations that had retained a commitment to social change. Their strategies had a number of elements in common. They all stressed the importance of strengthening women's material position: through micro-credit in one case, group-based savings in the others. They emphasised the need for cognitive change through organised training and informal discussion. Also, they sought to build up relations of solidarity between group members in contrast to the instrumental 'group liability' approach which motivated conventional microfinance organisations.

The women's narratives offered important insights into the processes through which individual empowerment translated into greater awareness of rights and greater willingness to struggle for them. They explained their past failure to act in terms of their fear of its consequences but also in terms of its inconceivability: 'We did not protest even where there was lots of injustice and oppression in the village. We were afraid of the chairmen, village leaders and members. Moreover, we couldn't even see any reason to protest. After all they are our village leaders, we used to honour them.' Or as another woman put it: 'We did not realise that we were human beings as well.'

The changes that have taken place since then occurred through a number of different routes. Women made a number of material gains through their savings, borrowing and training activities. These were by no means sufficient to allow them to leave difficult relationships but they did expand their scope for renegotiating them. They were less dependent on male earnings, more able to contribute to the household income and no longer had to rely on patron–client relationships that had provided them with some measure of security in the past but on very demeaning terms.

Change also took cognitive forms. The organisations in question offered practical training on livelihoods as well as opportunities for reflection and analysis. The awareness that the women gained through their interactions was transformative in its impact. They learnt to recognise the value of their unpaid contributions to the family and to demand such recognition from others. They learnt about arbitration and conflict resolution which in turn strengthened their capacity to make reasoned judgements rather than relying on given norms. They learnt about their status as citizens and what it meant to be an active citizen.

In addition, the women spoke of the value they attached to the relationships that they had formed through their group activities: 'One stick can be broken, a bundle of sticks cannot.' Group-based solidarity was purposively nurtured by the organisations through regular face-to-face interactions between group members, collective savings, periodic cultural events and participation in various forms of collective action to claim their rights and protest against injustice. In a society where women are expected to observe cultural norms of female seclusion, similar to those reported in Afghanistan, such public action represents a remarkable change.

Women used their newly developed capabilities to organise around a range of issues. Within the economic domain, they participated alongside men in struggles over unclaimed government land to which landless groups had legal entitlement but which had been forcibly occupied by powerful land owners. In the policy domain, they carried out the informal monitoring of government programmes for the poor, protesting against examples of corruption and unfair distribution. They had also become more active in the political domain, campaigning for pro-poor candidates during elections and, in some cases, contesting local elections.

When it came to injustices in the domestic domain, however, responses were more ambivalent. Women's groups took a strong stand against public forms of violence against women, including rape and acid attacks, and against a range of institutionalised practices, such as dowry and child marriage, which they regarded as the unacceptable face of patriarchy within the family. But in relation to actual instances of patriarchal injustice in their own lives or in the lives of women they knew, their approach was more conciliatory, marked by greater willingness to compromise.

One way to understand this disjuncture is in terms of the continued centrality of family in social life in Bangladesh and the near universality of marriage. Even if these women had managed to gain much more on the economic front, there is still very little social space in rural Bangladesh for them to set up their own independent households to escape abusive marriages. Most opted to remain within marriage, but renegotiate its terms.

Discussion of the Narratives

These narratives from Afghanistan and Bangladesh speak directly to the concerns of this paper. Firstly, they illustrate the variety of intended and unintended ways in which women's agency can be enhanced. The Afghan context offered striking examples of the unintended consequences for gender relations that have been generated by the rapid succession of regimes, with very contrasting views about women's place within society, as well as by the accompanying displacements from countryside into towns and neighbouring countries. Currently, purposive efforts on the part of state, donors and civil society to transform gender relations compete with the equally purposive efforts of conservative forces to resist such transformation. Such contestations had served to open women—and men—to the possibility of different ways of organising society and different models of gender relations.

In Bangladesh, a great deal of change has happened as a part of 'normal' development efforts, not necessarily intended to empower women. Nevertheless, the promotion of family planning and girls' education as a part of government policy, the emergence of new economic opportunities for women in the export garment sector, the proliferation of NGOs targeting women for various forms of service provision and greater exposure to the media have all helped to expand the associational possibilities and life choices available to women.

Secondly, even within the small and relatively homogeneous samples of women that were studied in the two countries, there was considerable variation in how they viewed the institutional arrangements that governed their lives, particularly the relations of family and kinship. Their views ranged from an unquestioning acceptance of the existing arrangements as 'given' by religion and culture to qualified criticism based on the perceived abuse of men's power to a more radical questioning of a system that gave men near-monopoly of power and decision making without holding them accountable in any meaningful way. While few of the women in the two studies came close to the full internalisation of cultural norms reported by Menon, neither did they turn their backs on the familial roles ascribed to them by their culture. What they sought instead was to renegotiate these roles in ways that respected their contribution to the family, gave them a voice in family affairs, expanded options beyond the family and challenged men's arbitrary use of violence. The pathways of change they sought were, in other words, 'path dependent', not crafted in a historical vacuum but shaped in important ways by inherited norms, values and institutions.

And thirdly, the two studies demonstrate how the different ways in which ideas about citizenship are disseminated in different contexts can influence the extent to which processes of individual empowerment translate into the ability to recognise and act on structural injustice. While women in both contexts are seeking to exercise a greater degree of agency in their own lives, it was the very different routes through which they became aware about their status as citizens in the two contexts that shaped the politicisation of this agency.

Women in our Afghan sample learnt about citizenship in almost accidental ways, only tangentially related to their association with development NGOs. Migration to Iran brought a number of them into contact with a very different kind of Muslim state, but it is worth noting that it was not differences in the practice of Islam in the two countries that featured most prominently in their narratives but differences in state effectiveness. Their time in Iran showed them what a functioning state looked like, its capacity to provide roads and electricity to its citizens and a police force that responded to women's complaints about domestic violence.

Within Afghanistan itself, while there were considerable restrictions on women's freedom of movement in the public domain, exposure to television and interactions with women beyond the confines of kinship through their economic activities and association with microfinance organisations had brought about a greater awareness about an emerging discourse of women's rights in the public domain. None of the women in our sample had ever sought to actually take their grievances to the newly established Independent Commission of Human Rights, but some viewed its presence as a restraint on men's misuse of their power.

The Bangladesh story was very different. Here women had acquired a greater say in their own lives and relationships as a result of the purposive strategy of organisations that also sought to transform them into active citizens. With the support of these organisations, women were able to use their knowledge of their rights as citizens to counter unfair verdicts issued by informal justice mechanisms within their communities, to bring to light the corrupt practices of government officials and to challenge the efforts of local elites to exploit their labour. Their successes on these fronts in turn strengthened their sense of citizenship, making it more difficult for men in their families and local power holders to violate their rights with the kind of impunity they had enjoyed in the past.

Conclusion

While the varying efforts of women in Bangladesh and Afghanistan to renegotiate rather than reject the patriarchal structures that governed their lives raise important questions about the universality of values of individual rights and personal choice, they also throw doubt on ideas about justice that are grounded in some unchanging and internally coherent notion of 'community'. If liberal arguments for justice are premised on false universalism, the cultural relativist case rests on an equally false essentialism. Both accounts need to be historically grounded.

Liberal ideas about individual rights did not always exist in Western societies. They emerged in the course of their transition from communities based on custom and relational constructions of personhood to communities based on contract and individualised notions of personhood (Fraser & Gordon 1994). While both Bangladesh and Afghanistan are societies in which family and kinship continue to play a dominant role in structuring social relations, they are also societies undergoing considerable change. In both contexts, we are seeing a gradual transition from doxa to discourse as some of the taken-for-granted aspects of social life are opened up to re-evaluation through the prism of alternative possibilities. In listening to the voices raised by women to protest against the unfairness of patriarchal structures as they have experienced them, we do not have to choose between an authentic local voice and an imported Western feminism. These are voices of protest grounded in local experience and articulated in local idioms in societies which are not hermetically sealed off from the rest of the world.

In her measured responses to Western claims to 'save' Afghan women from patriarchal oppression, first through invasion and then through development, Abu-Lughod (2002) raised the question that others cited have also raised: are emancipation, equality and rights part of some universal discourse of justice to which we must all subscribe? She suggests that there may be other values, such as closeness with family and cultivation of piety, to which women in different parts of the world may give greater priority: 'they might be called to personhood, so to speak, in a different language' (p. 788). While her concerns are addressed to the neo-colonial attitudes to Muslim women she has encountered among many Western feminists, the research cited in this paper reminds us that Muslim societies are not internally homogeneous: different pathways to personhood can co-exist within them. Gender justice surely requires societies that can accommodate these multiple pathways, the pious and the secular, the individual and the collective, without necessarily privileging one or negating the other.

In any case, the search for gender justice cannot be divorced from the larger question of social justice. Gender is not the only source of injustice in a society. Oriya Brahmin constructions of gender and family life position the women in Menon's sample as the privileged caste in an oppressive caste hierarchy in which men and women occupying the lowest position are deemed 'untouchable' because of the lowliness of their birth. The various practices that Oriya Brahmin men and women undertake to 'refine' themselves by regulating their contact with the outside world also represent their efforts to protect themselves from polluting contact with the lower castes. Women's active compliance with these practices serves to defend and reproduce both caste distinctions between the higher 'twice born' castes and the unclean lower castes and gender distinctions that see women's bodies as more polluted, and polluting, than those of men.

The fact that individualism in the *ontological* sense, the claim that a society is made up of atomised individuals and is no more than the sum of these individuals, has little traction in societies such as those discussed in this paper does not rule out the value of an *ethical* individualism, the recognition that certain basic rights and duties are defined in relation to the individual and rests on the equal humanity of all individuals (Robeyns 2003). A commitment to the fundamental equality of all individuals on the grounds of their common humanity is perfectly compatible with a worldview that recognises the connections between people, the socially embedded nature of their identities and experiences. It must also be fundamental to any understanding of justice.

Acknowledgements

Thanks are due to Professors Hilary Standing and Christine Koggel for comments on earlier drafts of this paper. The research drawn on in this paper was funded by the Department for International Development, UK.

References

Abu-Lughod, L. (2002) 'Do Muslim Women Really Need Saving? Anthropological Reflections on Cultural Relativism and its Others', *American Anthropologist*, Vol. 104, no. 3, pp. 783–90.

Barakat, S. & Wardell, G. (2002) 'Exploited by Whom? An Alternative Perspective on Humanitarian Assistance to Afghan Women', *Third World Quarterly*, Vol. 23, no. 5, pp. 909–30.

Basu, A. M. (1996) 'Girls' Schooling, Autonomy and Fertility Change', in *Girls' Schooling, Women's Autonomy and Fertility Change in South Asia*, eds R. Jefferey & A. M. Basu, Sage, New Delhi, pp. 48–71.

Benhabib, S. (1992) *Situating the Self: Gender, Community and Postmodernism in Contemporary Ethics*, Polity Press, Cambridge.

Fraser, N. & Gordon, L. (1994) 'Civil Citizenship against Social Citizenship? The Condition of Citizenship', in *The Condition of Citizenship*, ed. B. V. Steenbergen, Sage, London, pp. 90–107.

Joseph, S. (1994) 'Problematizing Gender and Relational Rights: Experiences from Lebanon', *Social Politics*, Vol. 1, no. 3, pp. 271–85.

Joseph, S. (1997) 'The Public/Private—the Imagined Boundary in the Imagined Nation/State/Community: The Lebanese Case', *Feminist Review*, Vol. 57, pp. 73–92.

Kabeer, N. (1999) 'Resources, Agency, Achievement: Reflections on the Measurement of Women's Empowerment', *Development and Change*, Vol. 30, no. 3, pp. 435–64.

Kabeer, N. (2011) 'Between Affiliation and Autonomy: Navigating Pathways of Women's Empowerment and Gender Justice in Rural Bangladesh', *Development and Change*, Vol. 42, no. 2, pp. 499–528.

Kabeer, N., Khan, A. & Adlparvar, N. (2011) *Afghan Values or Women's Rights? Gendered Narratives about Continuity and Change in Urban Afghanistan*, IDS Working Paper no. 387.

Kandiyoti, D. (1988) 'Bargaining with Patriarchy', *Gender and Society*, Vol. 2, no. 3, pp. 274–90.

Lister, R. (1997) 'Dialectics of Citizenship', *Hypatia*, Vol. 12, no. 4, pp. 6–26.

Menon, U. (2000) 'Does Feminism have Universal Relevance? The Challenges Posed by Oriya Hindu Family Practices', *Daedalus*, Vol. 129, no. 4, pp. 77–99.

Nedelsky, J. (1993) 'Reconceiving Rights as Relationship', *Review of Constitutional Studies*, Vol. 1, no. 1, pp. 1–26.

O'Neill, O. (1990) 'Justice, Gender and International Boundaries', *British Journal of Political Science*, Vol. 20, no. 4, pp. 439–59.

Robeyns, I. (2003) 'Sen's Capability Approach and Gender Inequality: Selecting Relevant Capabilities', *Feminist Economics*, Vol. 9, no. 2–3, pp. 61–92.

Unlocking Pathways to Women's Empowerment and Gender Equality: The Good, The Bad, and the Sticky

Patti Petesch

This paper brings together the concepts of social norms and innovation diffusion to assess two community development projects with gender targets. The projects failed to meet their objectives although they embodied leading global 'good practices' for community-based participatory approaches. In order to succeed, the projects needed to reach and empower poor women; however, they were located in contexts with significant gender inequalities and weak governance in one case, and with political conflict in the other. In such contexts, participatory projects with gender objectives likely require more strategic and longer term interventions than current community development models are allowing.

In the gender literature, stickiness is a bad thing. Sticky gender norms and power relations lock women into lives of subordination and isolation. In the innovation literature, by contrast, stickiness is the holy grail—it's the special quality of successful innovations that allow them to take hold and go to scale.[1]

This paper engages both concepts of stickiness, one being more political and the other more tactical. The two concepts are woven together to assess two international development projects that required effective local participation in

---

1. The author developed portions of the material presented here as background for Malhotra *et al.* (2009).

order to deliver the results being sought. In both cases, participatory approaches were being applied in challenging contexts and had poor outcomes. At the same time, both cases happen to feature some of our leading global 'good practices' in international development efforts designed to reach and empower poor women. The broad implications of using these approaches for assisting poor women everywhere are a fundamental consideration of this paper.

Grassroots participatory models, when they work as intended, reduce costs and improve the sustainability and coverage of projects.[2] Yet scholars and practitioners have struggled for decades with the fact that decentralized projects intended to benefit women often go awry and sometimes even harm women.[3] Which participatory approaches and when, how, and why they work as intended for women is still not well understood or demonstrated in evaluations. There is even less understanding regarding women in contexts that are remote and with deeply traditional gender norms or that are struggling with violent political conflict—contexts that characterize the two cases in this paper. My hope is that more systematic attention to the twin stickies of the political and tactical dimensions of interventions designed to empower women will point to better program designs and delivery.

Understanding Forces that Shackle and Unshackle

This section examines the concepts of sticky gender norms and sticky innovations. Both concepts borrow from similar sociological theories about the roles of culture and structures and how they interact to shape human behavior. Despite these commonalities, the gender and innovation fields feature quite different perspectives on the forces and strategies that bring social change.

The Hold of Gendered Social Norms

Gendered social norms embody a society's deepest values of what it means to be a 'real' woman or a 'real' man. Without the puzzle pieces of how gender norms

---

2. A review of 12,000 standpipes in 49 developing countries around the world showed that when national water agencies assumed maintenance responsibilities, the standpipes broke down 50 percent of the time; when communities controlled their maintenance, these rates plunged to 11 percent (Narayan 1995). For more recent evidence about the contributions of participatory projects to development effectiveness, see John Gaventa's excellent work at the Development Research Centre on Citizenship, Participation and Accountability (http://www.ids.ac.uk/go/idsproject/development-research-centre-on-citizenship-participation-and-accountability).

3. Mayra Buvinic warned over 25 years ago of gender and development projects that often 'misbehave' as economic objectives become sidelined during implementation due to gender norms surrounding women's roles and due to the welfare orientation and skill-set of many providers working on gender: 'These projects survive their financial misfortunes only because social or community development goals...take precedence over or replace production concerns when women are involved as project beneficiaries' (1986, p. 654). For another rich discussion of the diverse obstacles confronting women's roles in and benefits from participatory schemes, see Cornwall (2003).

function and constrain women's sense of self-efficacy and aspirations, one cannot make sense of why so many women around the world act in ways that undermine their own interests in their everyday lives. In some cultures, for instance, the shame and stigma of rape is so damaging to a family's honor that even the youngest of victims would know that she should never confide in anyone about such an attack—even though her shame and despair may drive her to suicide. In more modernized societies, gender norms surrounding women's roles and aspirations have the effect of steering talented women away from upper management positions.

Interactional explanations of inequality have been applied to shed light on the stickiness of norms even when their persistence no longer makes objective sense. The theory contends that norms and behaviors around group identities hold strong influence over interactions between social groups, including in circumstances where the attributes of the particular individuals who are interacting might not conform to those of their group (Tilly 2007). For instance, a woman may be the main or sole breadwinner in her household but she still shoulders the lion's share of household work and childcare and defers to her spouse on important purchasing decisions. Or engineering firms will continue to hire males over females because they have no experience working with women on their teams. Interactional approaches can enlighten us about how inequalities persist despite changing gender roles and the advent of progressive laws and norms that discourage discriminatory behavior and attitudes.

Cecilia Ridgeway's work (Ridgeway & Smith Lovin 1999; Ridgeway & Correll 2000, 2004) closely examines everyday social interactions between men and women to demonstrate how our unconscious beliefs about gender differences shape attitudes and behaviors virtually 'everywhere', shedding light on a core mechanism by which gender inequalities are perpetuated. Evidence from the field of psychology indicates that mixed-sex interactions automatically trigger thought processes which involve sex categorization and activation of widely held and deeply rooted cultural beliefs about men's greater competence than women's; and these background processes in turn disadvantage women in subtle and not-so-subtle ways as they interact with men, especially when the topic of the interaction touches on traditional gender roles (Ridgeway & Smith-Lovin 1999). Ridgeway and Correll argue that biasing against women is far more difficult to dislodge than race, class, or religious divides because social pairings between the sexes occur with much higher frequency and intimacy than between the other social group categories: 'gender goes home with you' in addition to permeating social relations in public spheres (2004, p. 512).

The Spread of Innovations

In his seminal work on innovation diffusion, Everett Rogers defines innovation as 'an idea, practice, or object that is perceived as new by an individual or other unit of adoption' (1995, p. 12). Innovation jargon and causal models can be found in studies about everything from drug marketing and new farming systems to communications technology and public health campaigns. Yet relatively little of the mainstream innovation literature is concerned with the problems particular to the inclusion of women in the design, use, and benefits of innovations.[4] Owing to space constraints, this section sets aside these important issues to highlight insightful lessons from the general literature on innovation diffusion.

Among the attributes that affect an innovation's rate of adoption, Rogers' empirical work repeatedly finds the *compatibility* of an innovation to be a key factor. The characteristics that make an innovation compatible refer to the extent to which its application is *consistent* or *competes with* local structures and norms. In a similar vein, Malcolm Gladwell explains 'the stickiness factor' as the particular qualities of an innovation that make it so 'practical and personal' that you are compelled to adopt it. The big lesson, according to Gladwell, is that nearly always there 'is a simple way to package information that, under the right circumstances, can make it irresistible. All you have to do is find it' (2002, p. 132).

The innovation field made major breakthroughs by breaking down the diffusion process into discrete phases with equally discrete adopter categories. In the early phase of diffusion, local opinion leaders play the central role in catalyzing early adopters to try out an innovation. In subsequent phases, when adoption rates peak and then decline (to create a non-linear s-curve for adoption rates), peer-to-peer interactions play a more important role than opinion leaders. What most often gets people to try out a product is seeing it being used or raved about by a peer. In short, word-of-mouth and demonstration effects are key for innovations to go to scale. But first, opinion leaders need to rev the engine.

The innovation field also recognizes problems of reaching lagging adopters, and research has uncovered important socio-economic and social capital differences that often distinguish different adopter groups. In his volume, Rogers points to numerous studies indicating that early adopters tend to be more educated, better off, and better networked than later adopters. He does not provide gender analysis, but one might assume that early adopters may tend to be male given these characteristics. These insights on the adopters help to shed light on processes that perpetuate social inequalities, including gender hierarchies, and buttress both equity and efficiency arguments for investing in additional measures to ensure that disadvantaged groups can access innovations and the opportunities they create.

---

4. Buré (2007) provides a useful overview of the literature on women's limited roles in science, technology, and innovation. With a focus on South Asia, Byravan (2008) reflects on women's frequent exclusion from formal opportunities to design, influence, and benefit from innovations, while their own important, but often informal, innovations often lack recognition.

Applying Both Stickies

The gender and innovation fields overlap in a few substantive ways. Both recognize the importance of power relations, social interactions, and social group differences. And both delve into the realm of the subconscious along with more overt influences on human behaviors. Nevertheless, the fields differ strongly in their outlook on the challenges faced, and hence the remedies required.

Theories of women's empowerment speak in the language of transforming inequitable gender relations. Change processes mostly transpire slowly because they are shaped by forces from the depths of internalized beliefs and norms, to the heights of society's most powerful structures. Sociologists primarily conceive of social interaction and social norms as constraining forces on social change. Diffusion scholars take an equally expansive view of social change processes, but from a position of far more speed and less explicit awareness of power relations. Stickiness applies to new ideas or ways of doing things, not old ones; and social group differences are perceived as targeting opportunities rather than constraints. Through systematic learning and tactical trials, seemingly intractable barriers can be surmounted. Ironically, the language of innovations has a more revolutionary feel than that of women's empowerment and gender equality.

With both concepts of what stickiness implies—one binding and one freeing—we turn next to the two case studies. The first case examines a healthcare program set in rural Ghana, and the second case presents experiences with enterprise development schemes in an urban community of Colombia. Again, these cases were selected because they embody today's most innovative approaches for advancing women's empowerment and gender equality at the grassroots. The two stickies provide useful prisms for understanding more clearly the qualities of participatory innovations that make them successful for women on the ground, but also vulnerable to derailment in challenging contexts. Both cases especially point to the importance of strong external partners who can adapt their innovative tactics to difficult local conditions in ways that enable meaningful local participation and strengthen women's agency.

The Navrongo Community Health and Family Planning Pilot

Rural populations of the African Sahel face levels of mortality and fertility that are among the highest in the world, with infants born in rural Ghana suffering a 50 percent higher rate of mortality than those in the country's urban areas. In poor and remote areas of the world, access to family planning has been proven to save the lives of women and their children and improve the well-being of families.

It is in the difficult setting of rural Ghana that our first case was implemented: an innovative grassroots pilot to work with village elites and mobilize village resources to strengthen demand for modern family planning methods and other primary healthcare. Launched in March 1994 by the Ministry of Health, the Navrongo community health pilot began in three villages of Kassena-Nankana District in northern Ghana.

Structured Learning about Local Structures and Norms

The Navrongo pilot employed a strong team of international public health specialists who began the pilot with careful field research, including qualitative assessments and a baseline survey to inform an impact evaluation. Rural women reported that they could obtain oral contraception from traditional birth attendants, but few did so. Various factors constrained their demand:

> Now if you say you want to limit your children, measles is dreadful and can even kill ten children at a go. So how can we limit the number of children? In Naga here, this problem still exists, so if you have five children, it is good for you to continue having children, because our eyes have seen in Naga how our children have been killed by this sickness. I have one wife, and if she is able to deliver the children, I will continue. I will not agree to *adog-maake* (stopping childbirth). I'm already suffering, but I will not agree to *adog-maake*. (Nazzar *et al.* 1995, p. 309)

Besides the scourge of measles, the fieldwork also revealed a high prevalence of other diseases, seasonal hunger, longer-term declines in rainfall, social status considerations associated with large families, local religious customs, bride-wealth traditions (and the woman's obligation to provide many children to carry on her husband's lineage), child marriage, and other local norms that strongly disadvantaged women and girls. On the service delivery side, as is common in other rural areas of the developing world, the formal healthcare system was largely inaccessible and people relied heavily on traditional healers.

The research also identified valuable entry points for the pilot. These included unmet desires for family planning, especially among women with several closely spaced births. With opportunities in farming disappearing, both men and women expressed appreciation for the potential benefits of having fewer but more educated children who could compete in urban job markets. Perhaps most importantly, the 12 chiefs in the Navrongo area expressed strong support for family planning. There are few details in the literature about how they came to hold these views, but one might surmise that they had been exposed to 'Western' ideas about family planning from earlier development interventions and from their business and political contacts beyond their villages. Their support, as the communities' gatekeepers and opinion leaders, was vital to ensuring that the healthcare services would be compatible and effective on the ground.

Drawing on these findings, the Navrongo pilot introduced two features. First, nurses were relocated from their inaccessible subdistrict clinics to small but functional village-based facilities. The nurses provided basic health services, of which family planning was only one of an array of services offered. Second, the project engaged chiefs, elders, and lineage heads as partners in the delivery of the pilot's outreach component. They served as local supervisors and publicly convened village meetings, or *durbars*, to disseminate project information and openly discuss health issues. The chiefs' engagement reduced the need for costly measures to raise awareness about the program and legitimized 'activities that might otherwise be controversial, thereby preventing needless conflict' (Nazzar *et al.* 1995, p. 313).

This is not to say that conflict was absent. Drawing on focus group data, Bawah *et al.* (1999) reported diverse tensions in gender relations associated with women's increased access to contraception. Both men and women described instances of marital discord, domestic violence, and tensions with other family members. Younger wives early in their childbearing years especially endured hardships. According to one young woman, 'If you discuss [family planning] with some men, they will get up and beat you' (Bawah *et al.* 1999, p. 57).

To protect and support women, and help men to understand better the benefits of family planning, the pilot team again enlisted the help of village chiefs and elders in educational outreach. Also important, when a woman reported abuse by her husband for using contraception, a team of male supervisors visited the household and called the community leaders' attention to the man's behavior, often persuading him to end the conflict.

The other signature component of the program, the redeployment of front-line healthcare providers from subdistrict clinics directly to villages, also relied heavily on community resources. At their own expense and labor, communities built compounds where community health officers could work and reside. The health staff then received additional training, motorbikes, walkie-talkies, and medical supplies that enabled them to provide ongoing doorstep family planning and other basic health services to women residing in remote locations and unable to reach the compounds.[5]

The impact evaluation covering the period 1993–99 demonstrated promising results. The experimental research design involved a control village where the program had not yet been started and three treatment villages: one village received just a community health worker, another just the community-outreach component, and a final village received both components. Drawing on panel data and econometric analysis, researchers found that the village which received both components saw a fertility decline of roughly 15 percent over the study period, outperforming the other three villages (Debpuur *et al.* 2002).[6]

---

5. The literature indicates that this component was very well received, but also created new pressures as demand rose for higher levels of medical care than could be provided locally.
6. See Debpuur, et. al. (2002) for discussion of factors besides contraceptive use that influence fertility rates, and the authors' other qualifications on program impacts.

Contagion and Mutation

By 1997 a favorable buzz about the Navrongo pilot was taking off. A well-equipped nurse in a village was outperforming an entire subdistrict health center, increasing by eight-fold the volume of health service visits (Nyonator *et al.* 2005, p. 26). District health officials began spontaneously to implement the program, but the transition from a pilot to a national program—renamed as the Community-based Health Planning and Services (CHPS)—happened so quickly that some of the most important design features of the pilot were lost; namely, the integral outreach components that secured the involvement of community leaders, and community participation, in support of the program. By 2003 the program was reaching all but 6 of the country's 120 districts; however, only 30 percent of these districts had the community outreach component (Nyonator *et al.* 2005, p. 31). Construction of community health compounds lagged even more. More recent evaluations, despite early warnings of poor performance, indicate that the government program continued to assign low priority to community outreach services and struggled with meeting implementation goals (School of Public Health 2009).

According to one evaluation, a major stumbling block was the lack of Ministry experience with outreach involving 'community diplomacy' and with understanding the local resources that communities themselves can and will mobilize under supportive conditions:

> Where CHPS operates [as intended], demand for services translates into resources for construction and other inputs. Community enthusiasm, moreover, offsets concerns about worker morale. But, these benefits of the program are not well understood in the abstract. Commitment to CHPS arises from experience with the program. (Nyonator *et al.* 2005, p. 32)

Innovative participatory processes can work well for women in difficult contexts, but they require an appreciation for the sticky gender norms that can often interfere, and the valuable role that trusted male gatekeepers can sometimes play in shifting mindsets towards greater inclusion. To work as intended, participatory tactics also require devolving real authority and resources down to local communities. Yet without the external support for the outreach component—the core tactical design feature that tapped into valuable local processes of transparency, inclusion, and accountability—this innovative health program was stripped of precisely the twin stickies that made the intervention compatible and tractable on the ground.

Building Female Entrepreneurship in a Cartagena Barrio

In this case study of participatory approaches with gender objectives we move to microcredit programs in urban Colombia and to smaller group-based participatory models. Microcredit that flows through small women's groups is the single biggest gender and development innovation of our day, and also one of the most widely used interventions for women in conflict-affected contexts. This case study, however, raises questions about the adequacy and appropriateness of this innovation for communities with continued insecurity and for external partners without a strong track record of effectiveness in these harsh environments.

Since the late 1980s, violence by several armed organizations has claimed the lives of tens of thousands of Colombians and displaced 3 million people, often to impoverished barrios (neighborhoods) on the rim of the country's major cities. Fleeing only with what they could carry in their hands, a large share of the urban displaced households has remained mired in poverty for years after displacement (Ibáñez & Moya 2007). Many women head these poor households, as husbands have been killed or remained in the countryside to join armed groups, work on farms, or try to hang on to their farmland.

This case study is set in Villa Rosa, a barrio on the outskirts of Cartagena that is home to approximately 700 people who have been displaced by the country's rural violence.[7] Villa Rosa was just six years old and still quite poor when the fieldwork was conducted in mid-2006. Women have great difficulty finding jobs or running their enterprises. One shop owner struggling to make ends meet explained that she cannot move on to something more profitable without an affordable loan. She had been turned down by the local bank 'because we live in Villa Rosa'—a place seen to be a war zone full of thieves and members of armed groups and drug gangs who are associated with the political violence in the countryside.

Investing in Women's Collective Self-help and Enterprises

Microfinance models vary but their signature sticky innovation is mobilizing women into small groups to manage small amounts of rotating credit at market or near-market terms. By channeling finance through groups of women who must vouch for one another and who can access additional credit when they demonstrate their repayment capacities, the innovation circumvents both the need for hard collateral, which is a great barrier for most women, and the sticky gender norms that surround women's restricted economic roles and lack of assets, and make it so that many economic development interventions almost exclusively target men.

As group-based microfinance schemes spread worldwide, credit alone proved insufficient for many poor women to realize material gains. Consequently, providers began to experiment with complementary investments in strengthening female entrepreneurship. Poor women around the world have now been recipients

---

7. The case study of Villa Rosa (a pseudonym) draws from nine detailed life stories and four focus groups with women of the barrio. The fieldwork was conducted as part of the World Bank's Moving Out of Poverty study, and this section draws on findings reported in Petesch and Gray (2010) and Petesch (2011). The data collection was not designed for a formal evaluation of the interventions.

of capacity-building activities in, for example, economic literacy, vocational training, and enterprise development and market support, with the hope that these inputs would help them to grow or diversify their often tiny home-based ventures and informal market activities. Some providers have also worked to organize poor women into larger enterprises and cooperatives to access inputs and sell their products on more favorable terms. Evidence of these advances could be found in the programs available in Villa Rosa.

Owing to an urgent need for income, several women of Villa Rosa reported participating in as many as a dozen different training and outreach programs. They said the programs built their skills and solidarity, and helped them to cope emotionally with the trauma of displacement and adapt to their new circumstances. Yet very few women reported economic gains from their participation in the schemes, and meeting the daily expenses of urban life remained a constant struggle for them.

The programs generally required the women to attend training and form their own local association, of which the women then might become leaders, treasurers, or workers in a shop, bakery, soup kitchen, or daycare. In their testimonies for the study, the women spoke highly of a local association with five members entitled Mis Esfuerzos (My Efforts). These women had received various training courses and a loan, and now run a cooperative variety store. They are hopeful the business might grow. Presently, however, it brings in little income for the women, although they put in long and sometimes risky hours. They are frightened by youth gangs and armed robbers who steal from them, particularly at night. Local women are sometimes afraid to come to their shop.

The enterprise initiative that local women reviewed poorly was an association of 20 women who received training in baking, business management, marketing, and customer relations. Together they launched a bakery offering sweet rolls, cookies, and empanadas. While the sales seemed to go fine, the women struggled with problems of poor returns and accountability. After dividing up the earnings, they barely had enough to cover bus fare to the bakery. There were also management problems, but few details were provided: 'I couldn't say anything. When I saw bad things, I had to stay quiet.' The same woman went on to report: 'My life improved because of my training, but it got worse because I didn't earn almost anything.' She felt exploited working from five in the morning until eleven at night, and she quit. She indicated that her husband is bringing in all of the income, for the time being at least, and she will not join any other economic groups.

Unaccountable and Shifting Power Structures

The women were also discouraged by their external partners who sponsored the enterprise schemes but lacked transparency and accountability. The women reported getting the runaround with documentation and organizational requirements. Promised loans and grants failed to materialize or arrived after extensive delays. Sometimes donor or government programs competed against one another for borrowers or community groups; or the external partners pitted different residents in the community against one another for scarce project funds. Most notably, significant community conflict arose out of the collapse of a housing assistance program. The initiative was supposed to help 100 households, but reached only three and led to bitter and ongoing divisions in the community.

If poorly conceived and implemented programs were not enough to stymie the women's economic initiatives, the ongoing violence in Villa Rosa was. Residents reported various forms of violence and crime involving guerrillas, paramilitaries, youth gangs, and unnamed armed actors. One woman indicated that she withdrew from running the housing association as a result of death threats, although it was a key local group helping women to access services. Perhaps most disturbing was the assassination of the community leader who had led the land invasion that established the barrio.

The barrio's leadership split into two factions in 2003, with some members of the neighborhood council having links to the paramilitaries and the others to the guerrillas. Testimonies described an ongoing campaign of intimidation; some community activists were forced from their posts, while others fled the barrio entirely. The women's external partners shut down their programs and also left the barrio.

The available evidence on the effectiveness of microcredit approaches for lifting women out of poverty in peaceful contexts is on balance promising but the gains are generally modest; there is little systematic information on the performance of microcredit programs in conflict contexts.[8] It is well documented that conflict often propels women into a more active economic role, and microcredit initiatives would be seemingly well positioned to build on and fuel this. Nevertheless, even in the best of circumstances, programs that seek to strengthen women's collective economic agency require external partners who can support local organizational capacities for transparency, inclusion, and accountability, and help their beneficiaries to anticipate and adapt to diverse and ongoing risks. Such risks are likely to be hallmarks of communities struggling to emerge from war. Instead, the women of Villa Rosa became saddled with poorly performing and unaccountable enterprises and partners who fled.

Concluding Reflections

Both cases featured innovative interventions that, in other circumstances, have surmounted sticky gender norms (the bad sticky) and ushered in new opportunities

---

8. See Chapter 7 of Banerjee and Duflo (2011) and Kabeer (2005) for their reviews of evaluations indicating that microcredit schemes can be very helpful for enlarging women's self-confidence and agency, but economic returns are generally modest. Kabeer stresses that the impacts of microcredit are contingent on community contexts; the characteristics of the women targeted, and program designs and providers (2005). She advises that these schemes have a poorer track record with reaching extremely poor women, although she specifically refers to skilled and experienced providers who sometimes have been successful with this.

(the good sticky) that gave many women greater independence and control over their lives. The contexts for these cases, however, were not compatible with participatory models in the absence of careful tailoring and effective monitoring measures. Because the Ghana project is rolling out slowly and unevenly, the lives of poor women and babies in large areas of the countryside remain at high risk. And because donor-sponsored enterprise schemes are delivering few economic returns in Villa Rosa, the women of the barrio have no cash to pay for food, electricity, rent, or other daily necessities.

The healthcare program went off track because the very component that made it sticky in both senses of the concept was disregarded. Without the community outreach and the chiefs' active engagement there were no means to raise women's and men's awareness about safe motherhood, healthcare, and family planning services, or to mobilize the resources necessary for communities to construct their own clinics. Participatory models require institutional capacities to devolve real authority and resources in ways that are inclusive, accountable, and transparent. Grassroots innovations that must work through government bureaucracies in order to go to scale also have to unlock the tactical measures required to shift these agencies' authority structures and mindsets in support of effective local participation.

The second case also failed to deliver meaningful assistance. For the women who gave long hours to training, organizing, and enterprise, their primary frustration was that the projects yielded few material benefits. Small and medium-sized enterprises are risky ventures in the best of circumstances. For these types of initiatives to take off in contexts with conflict and weak markets, providers are needed who can bring expert twinning of political and tactical know-how and more substantial resources than are currently being invested. These women needed more support to raise profits and strengthen their management capacities.

Nearly 400,000 rural women of Bangladesh participate in the Grameen Village Phone program, which must be the single largest female enterprise scheme in the world. In hindsight, the program is lauded for getting rural women in on the ground floor of a multi-billion dollar industry. Yet taking this leap was less than obvious in one of the world's poorest countries, in weak rural markets, in localities that by tradition put women at the very end of the line, and for a venture requiring heavy up-front investment. Grameen stacked the deck in the women's favor. The first 50 women selected to become cell phone operators all had strong repayment histories, but the eligibility requirements did not stop there. The first operators were also *already* running profitable businesses, literate, *and* residing in a home with electricity located in the center of their village (Bayes *et al.* 1999). In other words, Grameen did not pilot this promising opportunity in a remote context or with a group of poor and displaced women residing in an insecure barrio. Nevertheless, once rural women of Bangladesh demonstrated that they could manage their cell phone businesses, and very profitably at that, the eligibility requirements became relaxed and the program took off like wildfire.

Inclusive grassroots development approaches are innovative, and their sticky tactics can and do reduce costs and improve the sustainability and coverage of interventions. We still have much to learn, however, about the conditions under which decentralized, demand-driven projects can work well for women because of diverse gender inequalities and other factors in and beyond their communities that restrict women's initiatives. We also have much to learn about how to stack the deck so that many women can access great opportunities and not just modest ones that add to their heavy time and work burdens and bring few returns.

Scheming on the ground for poor women living in harsh environments remains an intensely political project, requiring savvy and experienced practitioners and a strong commitment of resources. We can sometimes help make projects more effective and salable by learning from and couching our activities in lessons about grassroots participation, male gatekeepers, social capital, adopter rates, community-driven development, and cost recoveries. Performance-based monitoring and experimental impact evaluations are also important to keep programs on track and take the learning forward. Nevertheless, very good information was not enough to prevent the Navrongo pilot from going off course when scaled up, and years of mixed evaluations of microfinance do not seem to be enough to put that approach on a stronger path either. Cornwall stresses that 'what is needed is not simply good tools or good analysis, but advocacy, persistence and influence' (2003, p. 1336). Fundamentally, women in deeply exclusionary contexts need politically shrewd and dedicated partners who will work with them to design and deliver the necessary tactics and financing, who will anticipate the ongoing risks of working to forge more equitable gender norms and roles, and who will not leave until their job is done right.

References

Banerjee, A. & Duflo, E. (2011) *Poor Economics: A Radical Rethinking of the Way to Fight Global Poverty*, Public Affairs, Cambridge, MA.

Bawah, A. A., Akweongo, P., Simmons, R. & Phillips, J. F. (1999) 'Women's Fears and Men's Anxieties: The Impact of Family Planning on Gender Relations in Northern Ghana', *Studies in Family Planning*, Vol. 30, no. 1, pp. 54–66.

Bayes, A., von Braun, J. & Akhter, R. (1999) *Village Pay Phones and Poverty Reduction: Insights from a Grameen Bank Initiative in Bangladesh*, ZEF Discussion Papers on Development Policy no. 8, Centre for Development Research, Bonn.

Buré, C. (2007) 'Gender in/and Science, Technology and Innovation Policy: An Overview of Current Literature and Findings', Innovation, Policy and Science Program Area, International Development Research Center, Ottawa.

Buvinic, M. (1986) 'Projects for Women in the Third World: Explaining their Misbehavior', *World Development*, Vol. 14, no. 5, pp. 653–64.

Byravan, S. (2008) 'Gender and Innovation in South Asia', avaialbel at: <http://www.esocialsciences.com/data/articles/Document1652009210.327572.pdf> [Accessed 11 May 2011].

Cornwall, A. (2003) 'Whose Voices? Whose Choices? Reflections on Gender and Participatory Development', *World Development*, Vol. 31, no. 8, pp. 1325–42.

Debpuur, C., Phillips, J. F., Jackson, E. F., Nazzar, A., Ngom, P. & Binka, F. N. (2002) 'The Impact of the Navrongo Project on Contraceptive Knowledge and Use, Reproductive Preferences, and Fertility', *Studies in Family Planning*, Vol. 33, no. 2, pp. 141–64.

Gladwell, M. (2002) *The Tipping Point: How Little Things can Make a Big Difference*, Little, Brown, New York.

Ibáñez, A. M. & Moya, A. (2007) *Do Conflicts Create Poverty Traps? Asset Losses and Recovery for Displaced Households in Colombia*, background paper for Moving Out of Poverty Study, Poverty Reduction and Economic Management Network, World Bank, Washington, DC.

Kabeer, N. (2005) 'Is Microfinance a "Magic Bullet" for Women's Empowerment? Analysis of Findings from South Asia', *Economic and Political Weekly*, 29 October, pp. 4709–18.

Malhotra, A., Schulte, J., Patel, P. & Petesch, P. (2009) *Innovation for Women's Empowerment and Gender Equality*, International Center for Research on Women, Washington, DC.

Narayan, D. (1995) *The Contributions of People's Participation: Evidence from 121 Rural Water Supply Projects*, Environmentally Sustainable Development Occasional Paper Series no. 1, World Bank, Washington, DC.

Nazzar, A., Adongo, P. B., Binka, F. N., Philipps, J. F. & Debpuur, C. (1995) 'Developing a Culturally Appropriate Family Planning Program for the Navrongo Experiment', *Studies in Family Planning*, Vol. 26, no. 6, pp. 307–24.

Nyonator, F. K., Awoonor-Williams, J. K., Phillips, J. F., Jones, T. C. & Miller, R. A. (2005) 'The Ghana Community-based Health Planning and Services Initiative for Scaling up Service Delivery Innovation', *Health Policy and Planning*, Vol. 20, no. 1, pp. 25–34.

Petesch, P. (2011) *Women's Empowerment Arising from Violent Conflict and Recovery: Life Stories from Four Middle-income Countries*, United States Agency for International Development, Washington, DC.

Petesch, P. & Gray, V. J. (2010) 'Violence, Forced Displacement, and Chronic Poverty in Colombia', in *Moving Out of Poverty: Rising from the Ashes of Conflict*, eds D. Narayan & P. Petesch, Moving Out of Poverty series, Vol. 4, Palgrave Macmillan, New York; World Bank, Washington, DC, pp. 192–247.

Ridgeway, C. L. & Correll, S. J. (2000) 'Limiting Inequality through Interaction: The End(s) of Gender', *Contemporary Sociology*, Vol. 29, no. 1, pp. 110–20.

Ridgeway, C. L. & Correll, S. J. (2004) 'Unpacking the Gender System: A Theoretical Perspective on Gender Beliefs and Social Relations', *Gender and Society*, Vol. 18, no. 4, pp. 510–31.

Ridgeway, C. L. & Smith-Lovin, L. (1999) 'The Gender System and Interaction', *Annual Review of Sociology*, Vol. 25, no. 1, pp. 191–216.

Rogers, E. (1995) *Diffusion of Innovations*, Free Press, New York.

School of Public Health (2009) *In-depth Review of the Community Based Health Planning Services (CHPS) Program: A Report of the Annual Health Sector Review*, University of Ghana, Accra.

Tilly, C. (2007) 'Poverty and the Politics of Exclusion', in *Moving Out of Poverty: Cross-disciplinary Perspectives on Mobility*, eds D. Narayan & P. Petesch, Moving Out of Poverty series, Vol. 1, Palgrave Macmillan, New York; World Bank, Washington, DC, pp. 45–75.

Empowering Children, Disempowering Women

Jan Newberry

The development of early childhood care, education, and development programs in Indonesia suggests unexpected linkages between democratization, empowerment, and neoliberal policy regimes. Despite the shift to grassroots organizing and to empowerment as a goal of development, in Indonesia there is tremendous continuity in the use of women's work to provide social welfare at the community level. Ethnographic research illuminates the impact on women's work and their own interpretation of programs to empower children.

Two years after the massive earthquake centred south of Yogyakarta in central Java, Indonesia, I visited a series of activists, educators, and governmental officials to ask about the appearance of early childhood care and development programs and their rapid proliferation in the area.[1] In the Yogya office of PLAN, the international child saving organization, my research colleague Nita Kariani Purwanti and I talked to energetic workers who had been sent from Jakarta to help in the reconstruction efforts. Here for the first time I heard the argument that the earthquake had made it possible for these early childhood programs to emerge. It was a dramatic statement, but then it had been a dramatic time for Indonesia. The massive earthquake had followed a year and half after the tsunami that had wreaked havoc in Sumatra and Aceh.

In fact, a series of natural disasters in Indonesia in the early twenty-first century seemed to manifest realignments in the political landscape as Suharto, authoritarian ruler for 32 years, was forced from office in the wake of the 1997

---

1. Ethnographic research in Yogyakarta began with original fieldwork in 1992. Recent research has included interviews with NGO representatives, early childhood care and education workers, local childhood experts, government education officials, and local women working in these programs.

Asian financial crisis, and democratization in its global, neoliberal form arrived in Indonesia. The development efforts of Suharto's New Order regime had been textbook modernization in the authoritarian mode—and strikingly successful. Democratization in the era of *Reformasi* at the turn of the century reformed development but in ways that showed significant continuity with New Order forms. The new early childhood care, education, and development (ECCD) programs that proliferated in the aftermath of the earthquake are an example of this. Known locally as PAUD programs for *Pendidikan Anak Usia Dini*, or Early Childhood Education, these programs represented the World Bank-inspired intensification of attention to child development during the golden age (*zaman emas*) from 0 to 8 (Departemen Pendidikan Nasional/Department of National Education 2002, 2006).

In the following, I consider how these new early childhood programs suggest unexpected linkages between democratization, empowerment, and neoliberal policy regimes in Indonesia. Approaches to empowerment and the idea of putting power into the hands of locals share an interesting and dynamic overlap with economic restructuring aimed at relieving the state of any role in community development and welfare through an emphasis on self-reliance (Harvey 2005; Sharma 2006; Swyngedouw 2005). Despite the shift to grassroots organizing and to empowerment as a goal of development projects more generally, in Indonesia there is tremendous continuity in the use of women's work to provide social welfare at the community level. At the centre of this consideration of empowerment is its relationship to women's work and the new desire to empower the child. What does it mean to empower children at the cost of exploiting women's labour?

Shifting Ground: Governing Women in Indonesia

As the interview with PLAN workers ended, we were invited to see some of the resources being distributed to the poor communities after the area earthquake. In the room behind the main office, we were shown piles of small, brightly coloured backpacks emblazoned with Ayo PAUD! or Let's Go, PAUD! Nearby there was a poster-sized development chart with pictures of children illustrating appropriate developmental stages. This poster was to be shared with local communities and community workers to illustrate more fully the various aspects of child development beyond the physical alone. This was in some contrast to the old health card that for many years was used to measure the growth in height and weight of children less than five years of age. Once a month, babies were weighed and measured, a healthy meal was served, and children who were failing to thrive were directed to the local health clinic through the justifiably famous integrated health post or Posyandu.

The Posyandu was part of a larger set of community-based, government-organized programs to promote social welfare in rural and poor urban communities.

Under Suharto's New Order regime, these programs were part of government-organized non-governmental governance (Newberry 2010). That is to say, these programs delivered community development inputs via local women whose organization was orchestrated by the government, but with little or no money. The New Order government was the epitome of a developmentalist state using modes of governmentality (Foucault 1991) to distribute rule through self-managing communities in order to guard and maintain the health of the population at large. And it was the unpaid labour of women that provided the workforce for these programs.

To understand the changes and continuities in these modes of governmentality in the era of democratization it is useful to describe the operation of the national housewives association, PKK, often translated as the Family Welfare Movement. This organization mimicked male-headed administration by placing the wives of local headmen as the leaders of the corresponding unit of PKK. The administrative bureaucracy in Indonesia began at the level of 10 contiguous houses, and extended through encompassment to the level of the nation. At its most local manifestations, these administrative units represented those living close to one another in neighbourhoods and rural areas headed by unpaid, popularly selected leaders.

Under the New Order, these local units of the national housewives organization were charged with holding monthly meetings to share governmental mandates and offering the monthly Posyandu health posts. These programs were begun in the 1970s and extended throughout Indonesia. Their growth can be traced to the push for the incorporation of women in development following upon the International Year (and then Decade) of the Woman in 1975.

In my initial research, I was concerned to understand how lower class Javanese women were stationed as neighbourhood volunteer cadres in charge of the health and wealth of their communities. A long history of productive work outside the home seemed to sit uncomfortably with a national ideology of the stay-at-home mother and volunteer social welfare worker for the state (Newberry 2006; Suryakusuma 1991; Wieringa 1993). And yet it was clear that, despite active resentment by many women, these programs were remarkably successful in organizing local health delivery. Infant mortality decreased as did the birth rate, as this organization was also responsible for delivering birth control to local women. Whatever their sentiments about the government programming, local women did feel it to be their responsibility to see to the sick and elderly in their community and to cooperate for community events. Still, given the fact that these programs were mandated by the New Order government, even if they were locally managed, I expected to see them end with the end of Suharto's rule. It was with some surprise that I found that the local units continued to function, although under different conditions.

In interviews, activists explicitly identified the 2006 earthquake as speeding the development of programming for children. Many programs emerged to deal with 'trauma healing' in young children. In a workshop I attended held for local relief workers, a young Indonesian educator proposed a child-centred approach to trauma. Its mixed reception indicated that placing children at the centre of programming was a relatively new idea locally. A year later, the situation had changed dramatically.

Child at the Centre

Child-centred approaches to relief in natural disasters are just one indication of a growing global concern with issues of child rights and child welfare. Typically dated to the 1989 Convention on the Rights of the Child, the growing inter-governmental and non-governmental priority given to the child marks a millennial return to the issues of children and childhood evident in scholarship and in people's daily lives. Concerns in North America with the end of childhood (Postman 1994) or its indefinite extension (Zelizer 1994) have been matched in the Global South with concerns regarding child soldiers, child labour, and child sex trafficking. In anthropology and other social sciences, there has been a growing call to produce child-centred research that gives primacy to the child's experience and voice (James *et al*. 1998; James 2007; Scheper-Hughes & Sargent 1999; Stephens 1995). The influence of empowerment approaches is evident in the call for child-centred approaches, but also in global inter-governmental policy towards the young. In 2002, children themselves served as delegates to a forum in advance of the World Fit for Children special session of the United Nations.

Attention to empowering the child is also reflected in the global emphasis on early childhood care and development, an initiative associated with the United Nations and the World Bank (Dahlberg & Moss 2005). The Consultative Group on ECCD, an inter-agency consortium that includes PLAN International, references both UN documents on child rights in early childhood (United Nations 2006) and Education for All, another global inter-governmental initiative associated with the 2000 UNESCO Dakar Framework. The use of the terms care and development in addition to education describes the comprehensive approach to child development advocated in these initiatives. As the Consultative Group on ECCD describes it:

> Framed by the UN Convention on the Rights of the Child, the ECCD field is interdisciplinary in its focus. It includes health, nutrition, education, social science, economics, child protection and social welfare. The ECCD field strives to ensure young children's overall well-being during the early years, providing also the foundation for the development of adults who are healthy, socially and environmentally responsible, intellectually competent, and economically pro-ductive. (Consultative Group on Early Childhood Care and Development 2011)

This is development multiply construed, as well as mimetically extended: the development of the child is understood as equivalent to the development of the country.

The arrival of ECCD programs in Indonesia has been rapid and extensive. As suggested, local activists and educators made the claim that the earthquake had sped the proliferation of early childhood programs in the area. That is, the earthquake removed not only physical structures but also bureaucratic and ideological obstacles to the entry of new programs. Indeed, local communities welcomed programming for the young as aid flowed into devastated communities. While the idea of ECCD has existed in Indonesia and the Yogya area since at least 2000, it was surprising how quickly ECCD/PAUD programs had spread through the area. As one activist noted in 2007:

> Since 2000 the PAUD program has experienced very significant progress, especially since it was proclaimed by the Directorate of PAUD in Jakarta. Articles concerning the young child were made official in that year. Now, the development of it is very fast, in the city of Yogya alone (not including the province) there are around 1000 PAUD programs. On July 21 of this year, there was a launching of 1000 PAUD programs in Yogya [province]...In fact the central PAUD Directorate (under the Department of Education) in Jakarta is in the process of accelerating the campaign...In this way, it is hoped the needs of children will be met. (Interview, 29 October 2007; author's interview and translation)

Much of the energy for organizing children's programming in Indonesia has come from the non-governmental sector, with activists and educators involved in rethinking education on the ground. In interviews these activists frequently made a direct connection between democratization and educational reform. Although Indonesia has long been the target of development work, the move to early childhood programs has coincided with the reorganization of the political and economic landscape globally. The shift towards neoliberal global governance has coincided with a wave of democratization begun in 1989. This shift has registered in moves to emphasize grassroots, non-governmental approaches to development. This, in turn, corresponds with the shift from women in development initiatives in the 1970s with their focus on equity in economic development and the importance of women's economic contributions towards gender and development approaches initiated with the 1995 Beijing conference on women. Razavi and Miller (1995) describe this shift and the advent of empowerment approaches, noting some of the contradictions in NGO and grassroots approaches that are not attentive to power such as neoliberal economic adjustment. In Indonesia, these shifts became locally relevant with the 1997 debt crisis in Asia, the introduction of neoliberal governance to the region, and the end of the Suharto regime and the beginning of the era of democratization.

One particularly salient example of the development of ECCD/PAUD programs in Yogyakarta derives from the work of a local NGO dedicated to the rights of women and children, namely the LSPPA (*Lembaga Studi dan Perkembangan Perempuan dan Anak* or Institute for the Study and Development of Women and Children). The LSPPA worked collaboratively with Australia's Agency for International Development (AusAID) and PLAN International to open the ECCD Research Center, which has served to train other organizations interested in developing

PAUD programs. The ECCD-RC has opened its own lab preschool and trained local women in the methods and theories of early childhood development.

This collaborative project between a local NGO, an international child saving organization and a government-run development agency is indicative of the kinds of governance arrangement emerging around early childhood programs. In many ways, this is nothing new in Indonesia. Indeed, the national housewives association's position as a quasi-governmental organization demonstrates the longstanding extension of state rule through non-governmental organizations of local communities. Yet, in the current context, this non-governmental govern- ance accords quite nicely with neoliberal dictates for the privatization of government programming and the flexible management of social welfare through outsourcing of functions. In this light, the tremendous growth in the NGO sector in Indonesia in the era of democratization poses some thorny questions about just how much citizen participation there is in empowerment projects of democra- tization. That is, do empowerment and democratization align strategically with the privatization and the individualization of welfare envisioned by neoliberalism (see Gupta & Sharma 2006; Sharma 2006)?

In the next section, the contradictions posed to women's empowerment provide a way to consider the continuity in governance across regimes in Indonesia. The question becomes: at what price to women's empowerment is the empowerment of children achieved?

Working Women

The emergence of ECCD programming in Indonesia has coincided not only with the reorganization towards democratic and decentralized non-governmental governance and empowerment approaches. It has also coincided with the expansion of the middle class in Indonesia, and with it the desire for private preschool and daycare options that had not been available on a widespread basis until recently. During field site visits in 2007 at private daycares and preschools, it was evident that these programs were designed for an upper middle-class clientele interested in status consumption of educational enrichment, such as English language classes, that are geared to produce achievement and improved class position.

The extensive use of preschool and daycare programs is a new thing in Indonesia. Even among the extremely wealthy, care of young children typically has been provided within the household by servants and family. The emergence of private childcare away from home has several implications. First, the expense associated with these private 'playgroups', as they are called locally, is significant. Families making use of these programs are quite well-to-do with private cars, drivers, and household help. Paying for preschool, then, is a symbol of middle-class arrival and not necessarily the needs of a two-income couple. Indeed, it was noted during interviews that these programs run for a very short time, a few hours at most, and they typically require a car to deliver and collect children. Consequently, it is unclear what support they offer to working women.

Whereas these private preschools did little to support working women, the public ECCD/PAUD programs depended on the work of local woman within their communities. As noted, there was an acceleration of PAUD programming provincially and nationally beginning in 2007. This dramatic proliferation in programming required a readymade structure to deliver it to rural and poor urban communities, and PKK and Posyandu provided this. The greatest growth in ECCD programs was actually through the same community-based organization used for the national housewives association. In other words, once again poor women were asked to deliver social welfare inputs voluntarily in their communities as their labour was conscripted to deliver ECCD/PAUD programming.

In a series of interviews conducted at local PAUD programs by my research colleague, Nita Kariani Purwanti, it was clear that PKK was a fundamental part of these programs, although it was not always the only influence. One of the fascinating aspects of PAUD programs is that they blur any clear line between health and education, and as a consequence there are many stakeholders in the programming. In fact, government learning centres and non-formal schooling programs, both under the Ministry of Education, are also important. Three programs are described below as examples of the paths to PAUD.

In the first case, a local PAUD program was started at the request of the local village head's wife. Although she began the program, it was organized and run by the women of PKK. The program itself was run for two hours three times a week on the terrace of the local mosque. This kind of schedule is typical, as were the costs at Rp$16,000 or less than US$2 per month. There are five teachers, all of whom have had training in the methods of PAUD and contact with both the professional organization for PAUD educators and with an association of allied PAUD units. This program is in a poor rural or peri-urban community at the edge of Yogya, and it demonstrates the PKK-run approach to PAUD. That is, the local leader's wife, head of PKK for the region, spearheaded the development of the program, and the PAUD teachers were supported with government training in their jobs.

In the second case, a young, educated woman became interested in making a playground in her local area and raised the issue with the local village head. Not long after, there were instructions from the local education board to begin this program as a 'PAUD pioneer' with support for play facilities. Although not initiated through PKK, there is Pos PAUD (PAUD post) associated with the Posyandu, and some parents make use of it to drop off children to be taken care of by health clinic cadres. As noted above, it is the local unit of PKK that typically hosts the Posyandu, and so the labour of these women must necessarily be involved.

In the third case, the PAUD program was only three months old. It was organized through another PKK-run program called Posdaya, or Family Empowerment Post, an example of the further integration of health and family services and their delivery in the era of reform. As one teacher noted, Posdaya is an organization that considers health, education and the economy (interview, 1 August 2009). According to the wife of the local headman, they received instructions 'that every *dusun* [village] must have its own PAUD so that the children, usually from poor families, can be educated even if they can't enter a playgroup' (interview, 1 August 2009). Here we see the explicit contrast between PAUD programs for the poor and the private 'playgroup' opportunities available for those who are better off. The teachers in this program noted that the idea to start a PAUD program already existed prior to the instructions from the government, a testament to the popularity of these programs at the moment.

The programs described here illustrate two things. First, there is the intensification and proliferation of community-based organizations aimed at supporting the poor and their families. Although the names and functions have shifted somewhat, there is great continuity in this non-governmental governance begun under Suharto and continued now in the guise of neoliberal, democratic reform. That is, the structure is given by the government, but the programming is delivered by locals, who may receive some very small monies, some training, and perhaps some other minor inputs. Second, PKK continues to function both in and around these programs, using women's 'volunteered' labour to staff and run these programs. Despite attempts to professionalize early childhood educators, this work is understood as different from formal work. Some of the contradictions implied in this positioning of working women as volunteers working for child empowerment are identified below.

Feminasasi of PAUD

In an unpublished paper from 2009, Indonesian education activist Sri Marpinjun outlined the causes of what she calls the *feminasasi* or feminization of PAUD. 'It appears that teachers in kindergarten programs [as well as other early childhood programs like PAUD] are considered to be doing the work of women when they teach school. This is what I call a symptom of the feminization of the PAUD' (Marpinjun 2009). She goes on to say:

> there is an assumption that PAUD is women's work, because it's best if PAUD is run by women. This is such a strong assumption by policy makers that they do not feel it's necessary to provide budgetary support for women who work as PAUD teachers. The mobilization of women for PAUD programs can trap women left behind in poverty because the national system of education is less responsive to them which is proven by the wages of the women who play a role in PAUD programming being far less than those earned by teachers from higher levels. (Marpinjun 2009; author's translation)

And there is ample evidence of this poor pay in the interviews I am drawing upon here. For example, the teachers from the first case described responded to questions about their pay in this way:

Respondent 1 (R1) [laughing]: A hundred [Rp$100,000 or about US$68].[2]
R2: 100,000…compared to how hard we work, it's nothing.
Nita: Just enough for gasoline, eh? (Interview, 13 November 2009)[3]

And in the third case described above, the PAUD teachers are not being paid at all. PAUD teachers often hold other jobs that earn wages. The work of PKK and now the work of PAUD seem to be grounded in an idea about women's willingness to volunteer labour and their natural abilities as organizers.

Yet it is clear that many women involved in PAUD programs contrast this kind of community work with waged labour. One woman commented that she took on work teaching in a PAUD program despite her own work as a kindergarten teacher because she felt that she had to because her local PKK group asked her to do it. While Sri Marpinjun begins by describing the work of kindergarten teachers, there is a felt difference in these kinds of work. One kindergarten teacher compared her work there with that of PAUD:

> In the kindergarten, I'm paid in a clear system, and parents [are] entrusting their children's education in my hand. In the PAUD, I'm working voluntarily, so if parents [are] complaining, for example, my way of teaching, I feel burdened. And since they also live in the same neighbourhood with me, and I'll feel wrong whenever I try to greet their children. For sure, the job is almost without benefits, but the burden is felt bigger. (Interview, 4 July 2009; translation Nita Kariani Purwanti)

It is PAUD's character as community-based non-governmental governance that extends and intensifies the 'burden' felt by women.

In interviews, two prominent Yogya feminists considered the causes and consequences of the feminization that Sri Marpinjun describes. The first of these activists, known here as Haryani, identifies the work associated with PAUD and PKK as deriving from government need to absorb excess labour, an argument that I have developed elsewhere (Newberry 2006, 2008, 2010). As Haryani says: 'This also relates to the problem of job opportunity in Indonesia; can the government answer this problem? To be PAUD tutors are like…well, you get a job rather than doing nothing, right?' (interview, 21 March 2011). Still, Haryani does not dismiss the need for early childhood programs, and neither does Indrawati, the other well-known feminist figure interviewed. She makes a case for the naturalness of women's role in early education—this despite the fact that her own son has followed in her footsteps to open a PAUD program for poor, rural children. Later, noting that men can indeed be teachers of the very young, she goes on to say that 'we—women—have to realize that men are not as skilful as women…because they are men' (interview, 27 December 2010). This pro-maternal feminism tends to run up against the needs for social justice now being framed in terms of the

---

2. The Indonesian national currency is the rupiah (Rp$). At the time of writing, 1 US dollar (US$) was worth Rp$8,500.
3. Unless otherwise noted here, interviews were conducted by Nita Kariani Purwanti and translations were provided by Ridzki Samsulhadi.

importance of democratic education for Indonesia's future. Indrawati herself notes that the feminization of education is less important than the feminization of poverty.

Haryani has more explicit concerns with the development of PAUD when it is not based on economic equity. 'There are many women who are "locked" inside the house. For example, the "smart parent program" turns out to be...it's the mother who should teach the children. Things like this hamper women to be active in the public domain' (interview, 21 March 2011; translation Nita Kariani Purwanti). Yet Haryani sees the positive potential for PAUD programs if they are managed as daycare centres that strengthen gender equity by allowing women to work. 'There should be male tutors too. Don't just replicate women's roles...it's meaningless' (ibid.). Here, the contradictions for women's work are quite plain. ECCD/PAUD programs do not function to help working women, and, in fact, they depend on the unacknowledged, 'volunteered' labour of lower class women.

By juxtaposing the words of noted feminist figures with those of the poor, local women offering the PAUD programs, the ongoing tension in the lives of Indonesian women is revealed. And that tension is between a sense that women's work is central, in fact crucial, to the health and wealth of local communities and the experience of modes of governmentality since at least the 1970s that organize development based on the exploitation of their work. In my own research, from its beginnings, I have argued for the acknowledgement of the contributions of women's labour as against its naturalization as an extension of women's duties as wives and mothers. The New Order made significant political use of the *ibu rumah tangga*, or the stay-at-home mother, in its domestication of women's labour within the home. To classify this labour as voluntary care is to remove it from the logic of capital and accumulation, and whether this is done in the name of authoritarian modernity and developmentalism or in the name of newly flexible and privatized neoliberal government and democratization, the issue remains the same. In fact, the apparent tension in the effects for women's work between private programs and community-based ECCD/PAUD programs resolves if both are considered as non-governmental programs delivered in a neoliberal regime. That is, both remove the state from responsibility in delivering early childhood enrichment even as it mandates its expansion through women's labour.

Empowerment?

I am not the first to note the unexpected synergy between the wave of democratization in the late 1990s and the globalization of neoliberal governance as an inter-governmental policy regime (Ferguson 2006; Gupta & Sharma 2006; Leve 2001; Sharma 2006). That is to say, grassroots approaches to empowerment seem to arrive at the same moment that global governance shifts to favour smaller governments, market incentives for governance, and shrinking social welfare budgets. The arrival of this approach in Indonesia hand-in-hand with democratization has meant that non-governmental solutions have been influenced by both neoliberal policy solutions as well as grassroots organizing for democracy.

This rather unholy synergy is evident in attention to empowerment. Empowering individuals to better themselves unintentionally extends neoliberal prescriptions for individualized solutions to social problems (Nagar & Raju 2003). This dynamic is also evident in the transnational push for attention to childhood by the World Bank (Evans *et al.* 2000; Penn 2002). The goal of empowering children through improved educational inputs for the very young child owes much to the drive towards democratic self-governance that is measurable, transparent, and accountable. In the case considered here, the extension of empowerment to programs to empower the child is evident in the development of ECCD/PAUD programs in the most densely populated part of Indonesia: central Java.

Christine Koggel (2007) notes, as does Mohanty (1997), the risk of neo-colonialism in development. And in this regard, it is interesting to note that the development of the child has long stood for the development of the colony, with savage, colony, and child collapsed into a single categorical invitation to intervention (Burman 2008; Cannella & Viruru 2004). This continues today. As Malkki notes, children are seen as symbols of world harmony embodying all of humanity. They function as a 'tranquilizing convention' in the international community that can serve to dehistoricize and depoliticize conditions (Malkki 2010). Yet if, as Tronto suggests, 'care, as a political concept, requires that we recognize how care—especially the question, who cares for whom?—marks relations of power and the intersection of gender, race, and class with care-giving' (1993, p. 169), then the case of ECCD/PAUD is one such intersection.

The effects of economic globalization are important frames for understanding how empowerment might function locally, as Koggel notes (2007). This argument can be extended to economic disparity *within* any locality. What is evident in the data presented here is that poor women are both targets and agents in local empowerment programs that demand their ready labour to offer early childhood programs. While this work is 'better than nothing', it is *still* work. And this is the same kind of work that women were given during the Suharto era of authoritarian modernization, when the New Order naturalized this as women's tendency to care for others.

Who can be against empowering children? Surely, this is a self-evident good to be embraced. Yet at what cost to the women who were once the targets of the very same empowerment rhetoric? In the case described here, Indonesian women's labour has been organized to deliver social welfare, first by an authoritarian modernizing regime and now by a democratizing, neoliberal regime; first, through women in development initiatives, and now through empowerment approaches. Yet there is a striking similarity across regimes in the work to be done by women for little or no pay and often in addition to other work. As the newly empowered child emerges in the new democratic landscape of Indonesia, what then of the wives, mothers, and sisters who work to make this possible?

Acknowledgements

My thanks to Nita Kariani Purwanti who served as interviewer, translator, and colleague for much of this work and Ridzki Samsulhadi who served as translator for some of the interviews. My thanks also to friend and mentor Professor Christine Koggel for her encouragement to continue thinking about empowerment.

References

Burman, E.(2008) *Developments: Child, Image, Nation,* Routledge, New York.

Cannella, G. S. & Viruru, R. (2004) *Childhood and Postcolonization: Power, Education, and Contemporary Practice,* RoutledgeFalmer, New York.

Consultative Group on Early Childhood Care and Development (2011) Available at: <http://www.ecdgroup.com/eccdinfo.asp> (accessed 1 June 2011).

Dahlberg, G. & Moss, P. (2005) *Ethics and Politics in Early Childhood Education,* Contesting Early Childhood series, RoutledgeFalmer, London.

Departemen Pendidikan Nasional (2002) *Acuan Menu Pembelajaran Pada Pendidikan Anak Dini Usia (Menu Pembelajaran Generik)* [*Learning Reference Menu for Early Childhood Education*], Direktorat Pendidikan Anak Dini Usia, Direktorat Jenderal Pendidikan Luar Sekolah dan Pemuda, Jakarta [Early Childhood Education Directorate, General Director for Out of School Education and Youth].

Departemen Pendidikan Nasional (2006) *Pedoman Penerapan Pendekatan Beyond Centers and Circle Times (BCCT) Dalam Pendidikan Anak Usia Dini* [*Application Manual for Approaching Beyond Centers and Circle Times in Early Childhood Education*], Departemen Pendidikan Nasional, Jakarta [Department of National Education].

Evans, J., Meyers, R. & Ilfeld, E. (2000) *Early Childhood Counts: A Programming Guide on Early Childhood Care for Development,* World Bank, Washington, DC.

Ferguson, J. (2006) *Global Shadows: Africa in the Neoliberal World Order,* Duke University Press, Durham, NC.

Foucault, M. (1991) 'Governmentality, Ideology and Consciousness', in *The Foucault Effect: Studies of Governmentality,* eds G. Burchell, C. Gordon & P. Miller, University of Chicago Press, Chicago, pp. 87–104.

Gupta, A. & Sharma, A. (2006) 'Globalization and Postcolonial States', *Current Anthropology,* Vol. 47, no. 2, pp. 277–307.

Harvey, D. (2005) *A Short History of Neoliberalism,* Oxford University Press, New York.

James, A. (2007) 'Giving Voice to Children's Voices: Practices and Problems, Pitfalls and Potentials', *American Anthropologist,* Vol. 109, no. 2, pp. 261–72.

James, A., Jenks, C. & Prout, A. (1998) *Theorizing Childhood,* Polity, London.

Koggel, C. (2007) 'Empowerment and the Role of Advocacy in a Globalized World', *Ethics and Social Welfare,* Vol. 1, no. 1, pp. 8–21.

Leve, L. (2001) 'Between Jesse Helms and Ram Bahadur: Participation and Empowerment in Women's Literacy Programming in Nepal', *PoLAR: Political and Legal Anthropology Review,* Vol. 24, no. 1, pp. 108–28.

LSPPA (Lembaga Studi dan Pengembangan Perempuan dan Anak) [Institute for the Study and Development of Women and Children] (2009) Available at: <www.lsppa.org>.

Malkki, L. (2010) 'Children, Humanity and the Infantilization of Peace', in *In the Name of Humanity: The Government of Threat and Care,* eds I. Feldman & M. Ticktin, Duke University Press, Durham, NC, pp. 58–85.

Marpinjun, S. (2009) 'Gejala Feminisasi PAUD', unpublished manuscript.

Mohanty, C. (1997) 'Women Workers and Capitalist Scripts: Ideologies of Domination, Common Interests, and the Politics of Solidarity', in *Feminist Genealogies, Colonial Legacies, Democratic Futures*, eds J. Alexander & C. Mohanty, Routledge, New York, pp. 3–29.

Nagar, R. & Raju, S. (2003) 'Women, NGOs, and the Contradictions of Empowerment and Disempowerment: A Conversation', *Antipode*, Vol. 35, no. 1, pp. 1–13.

Newberry, J. (2006) *Back Door Java: State Formation and the Domestic in Working Class Java*, Broadview Press, Peterborough.

Newberry, J. (2008) 'Double Spaced: Abstract Labour in Urban Kampung', *Anthropologica*, Vol. 50, no. 2, pp. 241–54.

Newberry, J. (2010) 'The Global Child and Non-governmental Governance in Post-Suharto Indonesia', *Economy and Society*, Vol. 39, no. 3, pp. 403–26.

Penn, H. (2002) 'The World Bank's View of Early Childhood', *Childhood*, Vol. 9, no. 1, pp. 118–32.

Postman, N. (1994) *The Disappearance of Childhood*, Vintage, New York.

Razavi, S. & Miller, C. (1995) *From WID to GAD: Conceptual Shifts in the Women and Development Discourse*, Occasional Paper 1, United Nations Research Institute for Social Development, United Nations Development Programme, Geneva.

Scheper-Hughes, N. & Sargent, C. (1999) *Small Wars: The Cultural Politics of Childhood*, University of California Press, Berkeley.

Sharma, A. (2006) 'Crossbreeding Institutions, Breeding Struggle: Women's Empowerment, Neoliberal Governmentality, and State (Re)formation in India', *Cultural Anthropology*, Vol. 21, no. 1, pp. 60–95.

Stephens, S. (1995) *Children and the Politics of Culture*, Princeton University Press, Princeton.

Suryakusuma, J. (1991) 'State Ibuism: The Social Construction of Womanhood in the Indonesian New Order', *New Asian Visions*, Vol. 6, no. 2, pp. 46–71.

Swyngedouw, E. (2005) 'Governance Innovation and the Citizen: The Janus Face of Governance-beyond-the-State', *Urban Studies*, Vol. 42, no. 11, pp. 1991–2006.

Tronto, J. B. (1993) *Moral Boundaries: A Political Argument for an Ethic of Care*, Routledge, New York.

United Nations (2006) General Comment 7, Implementing Child Rights in Early Childhood (40th session, 2005), UN Doc. CRC/C/GC/7/Rev.1.

Wieringa, S. (1993) 'Two Indonesian Women's Organizations: Gerwani and PKK', *Bulletin of Concerned Asian Scholars*, Vol. 25, no. 2, pp. 17–30.

Zelizer, V. A. (1994) *Pricing the Priceless Child: The Changing Social Value of Children*, Princeton University Press, Princeton.

Implications of Customary Practices on Gender Discrimination in Land Ownership in Cameroon

Lotsmart Fonjong, Irene Fokum Sama-Lang and Lawrence Fon Fombe

Africa, before European colonization, knew no other form of legal system outside customary arrangements. Based on secondary sources and a primary survey conducted between 2009 and 2010 on the situation of women and land rights in anglophone Cameroon, this paper examines the grounds for discrimination in customary laws against women's rights to land in the context of legal pluralism, and discusses the implications of this custom of gender discrimination. In drawing from Cameroon as an exemplar, it concludes that the strong influence and impact of customs on current land tenure systems have global implications on women's land rights, food security and sustainable development, and that gender equality in land matters can be possible only where the critical role of ethics is recognized in pursuit of the economic motive of land rights.

Introduction

In most traditional economies, customary laws uphold the principle of patriarchy in which girls and women are discriminated against from birth and socialized to live a life of male subordination throughout, either as daughters, sisters, wives, or widows. This leaves women with little power in decisions that affect their lives. The literature on women and land in sub-Saharan Africa and part of Southeast Asia is generally pessimistic on the possibilities of women owning land through inheritance. Palmer (2002), for example, points to the literature on gender and land rights, indicating the barriers and stiff resistance from stakeholders on issues of land rights, despite many years of lobbying and evidence from economic research and analysis of the role women play in all spheres of life. Land distribution and tenure in sub-Sahara Africa is still governed and managed by local customary tenure systems of rights (UNRISD 2006, p. 3).

Land remains a principal yet contentious factor of production in most developing economies of Africa, South America and Asia. Over time the land questions have shifted towards issues surrounding access to and control of land. Security of tenure not only affects women but also entire communities some-times forced to migrate in search of space for settlement or cultivation due to 'demographic pressure, wars and conflicts' (Friis & Reenberg 2010). They may also move in search of new economic opportunities, which can serve as alternatives to land. Access to and control of land by the community—men and women and by strangers—is thus guided by a set of principles which differ slightly among communities and which have also changed over time.

Diaw (1997), in his historical analysis of land rights in Southern Cameroon, identified two principles that define the types of rights over land: the ax rights and the usufruct rights principles. The ax, otherwise known as the blood principle, gives collective rights to the community over delineated land. Within this principle exists the usufruct right or territorial rights obtained by an individual after clearing a piece of land (sign of occupancy). Such description by Diaw, which can be observed elsewhere, brings to the forefront the delicate issues of customs and statutes that individuals and particularly women have to constantly negotiate over land.

For women, there are two ways in which most can acquire land: either through family bond (users' rights) or through transactions (purchase, lease, rent). Yet within the current global context of land scarcity and land grabbing, the demand has become more competitive, thereby generating diverse struggles. It has also complicated the prospects of women accessing land in predominantly patriarchal settings, where colonization and other dynamics have tilted the gender balance in favour of the males. As Fissiy (1992, p. 75) observes, in Cameroon the rise in the profile of coffee as a cash crop in early post-independent anglophone Cameroon together with the launching of 'Operation Green Revolution' in 1973 that intended to convert peasant farmers into 'bourgeoisie planteurs', led men to embrace coffee and cocoa cultivation for which they confiscated fertile lands previously cultivated by their wives or sisters. This was also the experience of Native Americans whose lands were confiscated by European settlers as a result of changes in economic and social dynamics.

Women's unsecured land tenure rights influence the way they use landed resources. They are less likely to invest time and resources or adopt environmentally sustainable farming practices on land they do not own or control or from which they may soon be displaced. For example, with the introduction of coffee cultivation in Bamenda by the Farms Office in Buea in 1922, women began to lose control over fertile fields as they were forced to move to marginal lands without being served quit notice(s). Fallow periods were forced to be shorter as land for their subsistence agriculture became scarcer. These lands rapidly became barren as a result of overuse (Kaberry 1959).

Data for this paper have been extracted from an ongoing study on women's land rights in Cameroon, and it is discussed alongside similar issues raised in the literature. Cameroon is a Central African country with a rich colonial experience that has significantly influenced customary practices in land matters. Anglophone Cameroon, for instance, sustained its very powerful traditional institutions which were allowed to operate during colonial times through British indirect rule, which encouraged the natives to participate in local governance and land management.

The Research Problem

Gender discrimination in land ownership in Cameroon has remained persistent in spite of the fact that the nation's Constitution, land ordinances, and other international instruments that Cameroon has ratified and domesticated gives women rights to property, including land. Despite women's triple roles (reproductive, productive and community) and the fact that their contribution to development is directly tied to land, it is still difficult for women to own land, particularly under the current pluralistic legal context governing land tenure. Thus, one finds a situation where customary practices seem to dominate the business of land ownership. The outcome, therefore, is the unwarrantable situation in which women's rights to land are not only violated but also their contribution to poverty reduction, food security and natural resource management is also negatively affected. Ironically, women are not the sole victims; humanity as a whole suffers. This is apparently the outcome of Mufeme's (1998, p. 5) admission that post-colonial African states have not done enough 'to change both the traditional and colonial heritages with regard to land and gender inequality'.

To address these serious issues this paper examines the arguments of customary laws vis-à-vis women's inheritance land rights in interrogating the state of gender-based inequalities in land tenure rights under customary practices in traditional economies such as Cameroon. It further explains the limits of gender-neutral statutory laws in the protection of women's rights and discusses the ramifications of women's unsecured tenure in contributing to poverty and impeding sustainable development.

The Context of Women Land Rights

According to Buchanan and Gunn (2007), basic human rights as set by the UN charter have no hierarchy. Gender discrimination in land ownership thus has no legal basis in most national constitutions, and laws do not recognize this form of discrimination. For example, the 1996 Constitution and the 1974 Land Ordinances of Cameroon are gender neutral. This Constitution in its preamble upholds that: 'We, people of Cameroon, declare that the human person, without distinction as to race, religion, sex or belief, possesses inalienable and sacred rights.' It goes on further to guarantee the right of every individual (women included) to own property by stating that 'ownership shall mean the right guaranteed to every person by law to use, enjoy and dispose of property'. There is therefore no legal basis, judging from the fundamental domestic laws, why women should be discriminated against in land ownership.

The same Constitution further affirms Cameroon's attachment to the principle of equal rights and 'to the fundamental freedoms enshrined in the Universal Declaration of Human Rights, the Charter of the United Nations, The African Charter on Human and Peoples' Rights, and all duly ratified international conventions'. Women's property rights in Cameroon are consequently upheld and protected by: the Constitution; the United Nations Declaration of Human Rights, particularly by Article 17 on the right to own property; and the African Charter on Human and Peoples' Rights, particularly in Articles 18 (3), 19 and 21 which point to the fact that no one shall be discriminated against or deprived of the rights to dispose of natural resources. Article 16(h) of CEDAW requests land tenure reforms to ensure women's property rights during and after marriage. It thus raises ethical issues when these provisions are publicly flouted by obnoxious customs and those involved, with state officials sometimes serving as accomplices or hiding behind custom, perpetuate what Whitehead and Tsikata (2003, p. 103) call 'elite-serving state power'. Odhiambo (2011) has also documented the same dominant effects of custom in favour of male inheritance and the lack of gender-sensitive family laws in Kenya, while Lind (2006) argues that even where women are entitled by statute to own land in India, social and religious factors prevent many women from doing so.

Methodology

A triangulation method was used in data collection consisting of fieldwork with reliance on questionnaires, interviews, and focus-group discussions in nine localities selected in 2009. This combination of methods enabled the researchers to capture valid and reliable data on key issues relating to gender, culture and land. The sample size of 2,205 participants included 80 per cent women and 20 per cent men from all socio-economic, political, demographic and ethnic representations. In addition to this sample, we identified and conducted interviews and focus-group discussions with leading women advocates, human rights NGOs, and traditional and administrative authorities. The process was facilitated by some 16 trained research assistants.

The target population was first stratified into male and female, with administration of the questionnaire ensuring that 8 out of every 10 randomly selected respondents were women. A variety of questions/issues were addressed pertaining to customs, land ownership, land use/management and poverty. Interviews were conducted with key actors (traditional rulers, women group leaders, administrative officers, parliamentarians (MPs) and mayors) who are directly or indirectly linked to land in order to corroborate information collected and elucidate different perspectives from respondents. Interviews and focus-group discussions offered insights on issues raised by respondents in the questionnaires and in the literature.

Customary Laws and Women's Land Rights in Cameroon

Statutory laws seem to exist more in theory, and customary law functions as the 'living law', which does not give equal rights and privileges to men and women. Aluko and Amidu (2006) argue that the complexity of land tenure in Nigeria is the result of the co-existence of several systems—customary, Islamic influence or state—none of which is completely dominant. This legal pluralism causes a degree of uncertainty about land rights, particularly for vulnerable groups, like women. That is why in the case of Cameroon, Goheen (1988, p. 90) argues that the 1974 Land Ordinances did not effectively encourage agricultural development but rather contributed to growing land scarcity and conflict; caused by the fact that both customary practices and Ordinances are not reconciled with each other. Customary communities in Cameroon, for example, do not talk in terms of national, private or state land but instead talk of communal, family and personal land.

Communal land belongs to a given ethnic community acquired either through first settlement or conquest and is managed by traditional rulers. Changes in ownership and use of common property affect households and communities differently according to their status on such property. In relation to Kenya, Karangathi (2005) stresses that changes in the use of common land have more impact on landless people such as pastoralists who depend heavily on common land resources for pasture and on women-headed households with limited economic opportunities. Family land is that part of communal land to which ownership has been conferred to a given family for settlement, cultivation or both. Rights over family land are inherited upon death by a male blood relation and transmitted from generation to generation through the son's line.

Privately acquired land is land owned by an individual with or without title and which has been acquired either through purchase, gift or lease. Ebi (2008) argues that it is difficult for personal land to be truly considered the exclusive private property of an individual in a typical traditional context because the upbringing of a child before he grows up to acquire a piece of land usually involves contributions and support from the family and its members. Women as wives (whether or not married under native laws and custom) find it difficult to assert their rights over such land, particularly in rural areas. Just as private ownership might create opportunities for women to own land through purchase, it nonetheless provides fertile ground for the exclusion of women and widens the gender inequality because of land grab and women's vulnerable financial status. Razavi's (2005) study complements this observation as in the case of women in sub-Saharan Africa, where the introduction of modern forms of property titling has instead undermined women's land claims. That is, where land reform has been accompanied by individually registered titles, women have often lost traditional customary claims to land while men's claims have been strengthened.

Customary laws are basic regulations governing the acquisition, management and transfer of landed property within a given ethnic community derived from the native laws, customs and sometimes religious practices of a community. Cotula *et al.* (2004, p. 2) describe customary land tenure as 'characterized by its largely unwritten nature, [and] ... based on local practices and norms, and is flexible, negotiable and location specific'. Reflecting on these characteristics, Njoh (2002) asserts that in the pre-colonial days land tenure was based on indigenous customary laws within purely traditional systems where the occupiers of native lands were no less than trustees who wielded merely the right of use without power to alienate. The notion of trustee is unlikely to exist today with the introduction of the market economy in which land is bought and sold, and with the advent of sedentary life.

Broadly speaking, customary practices differ across communities and coun- tries since these customs represent the identity of a people. Women's rights to land under customs are fragile, transient and unsecured. These practices are enforced by traditional rulers and male-dominated traditional councils and, at times, are recognized by statutory laws as in the case of Uganda, Kenya and South Africa, where customary land tenure has been incorporated into the Land Act. In Cameroon, customary marriages are recognized by the Civil Status Ordinance (Section 49 of Ordinance no. 81-02 of 29 June 1981), which requires these marriages to be registered after customary procedures.

Most of the studied customary communities surveyed reclassified women into: wives, single/unmarried daughters, younger and older widows, indigenes, and non-indigenes (with unequal access to land). Gray and Kevane (1996) believe that senior wives have stronger land rights than junior wives, insinuating that these rights increase with years in marriage. Female non-indigenes have more rights than their indigenes counterparts in communities like Kom where the Fon believe that land can be sold to strangers, while denying their own women this same right and opportunity. In relation to Nigeria, Aluko and Amidu (2006) note that marriage is used as a determining variable by which women and men access land under the customary tenure system. In the case of women, access to land very much depends upon age and marital status (including type of marriage and success of the marriage), whether they had children (including the number and sex of those children) and their sexual conduct. Women's land rights cannot continue to be defined by their relationship to men, because men and women have different perceptions of and interests in land.

Customary Fallacies of Gender Discrimination in Land Rights

Customary laws uphold tenaciously to patriarchy, which is the belief in a world where men dominate and control women. Celebrations accompany the birth of a male baby while hostility may be the reaction to the birth of a girl. This is reinforced by the practice of selective abortions of female foetuses and female infanticide in countries such as China. Kambarami (2006) reckons that patriarchal attitudes are bred in the family and village circles through a process of socialization, whereby the young are made to accept sexually differentiated roles. They learn that it is the natural way of life for men to dominate women and own all landed property, while the women can only work on the property. The lack of land ownership amongst women can therefore be attached to the fact that women grow from girls to know that they do not have a say in land. Patriarchy thus provides the basis for the emergence of a number of related fallacies by advocates of customary practices to explain why women should not have land rights in matrilineal and patrilineal societies. Be it from the marriage, chattel, levirate or remarriage standpoints, these fallacies portray the notion of power differences within the backdrop of chauvinistic ideologies with the sole objective of devaluing women's work or achievements.

According to the *marriage fallacy*, women, and particularly daughters, should not inherit their father's landed property because they will eventually get married. A woman's inheritance rights will amount to carting away family land to her husband's family, thereby reducing the available land of her maternal family (Ngwafor 1993, p. 199). Guivant (2001) reports similar reasons for the exclusion of daughters from inheritance of land in Brazil.

The argument gathered from field interviews in Cameroon is that the girl's identity is 'elsewhere' because, as they put it: 'she is a pilgrim': 'she will have land where she will get married'. Proponents of this myth consider it inconceivable and maintain that

> It is not healthy for a woman for that matter to continue to have influence over property in her maternal home once married, because not only will she run into conflicts with other women in this compound, but this also runs counter to normal reasoning and customary ethics.

Such is argued by a traditional ruler from Cameroon. However, male children born out of wedlock by these single mothers tend to have more land rights and arguments over family land than their mothers in most of these communities.

Closely linked to the remarriage myth is the myth of *the family name and remarriage*. Opinions expressed during interviews and focus-group discussions converge towards the fact that women are not always stable in marriage and cannot be trusted with such family valuables like land. This view holds that if a married woman (wife) is given tenurial rights over her husband's land, upon the death of a husband or divorce she will go with the land, thereby depleting the patrimony of her husband's lineage (Ngwafor 1993). An interview with the Paramount ruler of the Aghen (Cameroon) revealed that the fear of losing family land to a stranger as a result of a widow remarrying, particularly out of the community of the late husband, complicates the chances of women inheriting land. A similar view was also expressed by 2.7 per cent of all the respondents (41.5 per cent) who were against women's inheritance rights on the ground that women are not worthy to be entrusted absolute control over land in the absence of a man. Rünger (2006), however, holds that marriage has no effect on the property of spouses in Ghana because customary law permits couples to maintain their separate identities and are seen in theory as two separate individuals. He justifies this claim by arguing that the wife during marriage 'does not in a strict sense become a part of the customary family of the man and the converse is also true for the husband' (Rünger 2006, p. 6).

The 'woman as property' fallacy assumes that women have long been considered as part of a man's wealth and property. A man's status in society was defined by his number of wives and his credit-worthiness by the number of potential daughters he can give into marriage, argues a key informant from the North West Region. This belief is associated with the notion of bride-price, which is deeply rooted in customary marriage. Ngwafor (1993, p. 197) reckons that a customary wife is regarded as the property of her husband once bride-price has been paid. As such, a chattel cannot beget chattel no matter her financial contributions towards the acquisition of such immovable property. Upon divorce or the death of her husband, she cannot lay claim on any such property. Moreover, the manner in which the bride-price is determined in some North and South West communities sustains this viewpoint. In these communities, bride-price is calculated based on the beauty, age, level of education, character and virginity of the girl. Upon divorce, the girl's family is expected to refund the bride-price for the divorce to be valid, although this is contrary to the written law. Customary marriages thus make women additional property for their husbands and make her vulnerable in the bid for land and property.

The Western concept of marriage or remarriage today goes slightly contrary to the traditional views postulated by the *levirate marriage* argument. Most Cameroonian communities surveyed hold the view that marriage is a union between two families and not two individuals. Customarily, a widow is expected to be inherited by a brother or close relative, who also inherits the property of the diseased husband. Levirate marriages are seen as possible options to secure property, as also reported in Senegal by Platteau *et al.* (2005). In customary Rwanda, levirate marriages served as an opportunity for continuity, as even children born in such marriages belong to the deceased husband (Burnet n.d.).

This thus creates no room to think about women owning land. However, the widow may be allowed to continue cultivating the portion of land which she occupied while her husband was alive, if she decides to stay within his family and raise her children. But as the chief of Bangem (Cameroon) insisted, she is not allowed to carry out any major transaction or investment on the land without authorization from the family of her late husband, or have an affair with a non-relative. The above discussion indicates that the plight of a woman in customary Cameroon begins with the search for an identity. Considered a pilgrim both in her maternal and marital home, she is in a weak bargaining position over land, consequently violating her constitutional rights to property which her male counterparts enjoy. Yet narrowing the argument only to the violation of rights while neglecting women's economic interests can be misleading in that men and women have different interests in controlling land. In Cameroon, women conceptualize land from a social dimension, placing emphasis on human capital, while men, on the other hand, regard land as economic value. What is needed is a paradigm shift in customary philosophy of women and in land matters to accommodate gender interests in land holding. This shift is possible only where customary institutions are accountable to their subjects, given that women in all cases make up the majority of the population. Ribot (2002) argues that accountability is a non-negotiable requirement in local governance that claims to truly represent the interests of its community. It thus calls for women and other interest groups to be represented in local institutions (Woodhouse 2003, pp. 1717–18) despite the difficulty of accepting women into key customary institutions in Africa.

Implications of Customary Laws on Low Land Registration by Women

One would have expected statutory instruments to provide more avenues for women to access land rights by diminishing the power of customary norms. Nevertheless, this is not the case in Tanzania, where the 1995 National Land Policy reinforces these customs by upholding that inheritance of clan family land and land between husband and wife shall not be subjected to legislation outside customary laws. Gender-neutral statutes in Cameroon, which provide opportunity for women to register and obtain security of tenure, still face resistance from customs and attitudes.

The findings highlight a disconnection between statutory land registration and women's interest in owning land. Be it among urban or rural women, the majority are unaware of the provision of statutory laws that give them rights over land. Even among the few who claimed to be aware of the law, less than 30 per cent of those surveyed across all categories have attempted to exploit the law and to apply for land certificates. The reasons advanced for this low interest in land registration centre on fear and ignorance, which has been translated to loyalty to obnoxious customary practices and the lack of an enabling administrative environment to facilitate registration. Generally, land registration information is limited; the process is long, costly and complicated for the average, poor and illiterate woman to follow.

Moreover, the Land Consultative Board in charge of land registration in Cameroon is not gender friendly. It is predominantly male and, although a public instrument, most of its members still hold tight to customary beliefs. The literature on land registration in Africa suggests that the procedure for obtaining formal land titles does not actually offer a better alternative to the traditional system. The process is still dominated by men, just as in the traditional councils where customary laws are applied. The general consensus seems to point to the fact that the arrangement of and relationships between institutions that uphold registered property rights are part of a greater structure which excludes the poor and women from exercising their legitimate rights. Moore and Meinzen-Dick (2008) believe that individual land ownership in this case benefits the tenure security of a privileged few who are able to privatize land in their name, but it generally results in the dispossession of large numbers of poorer land users who previously had access to these resources. These are serious concerns added to the corruption of public land officials who referred to land as the 'black man gold' where they mine their riches. In fact, where sufficient information and possibilities for land registration do not exist, it becomes unethical to use registration as the basis of ownership because many women and rural dwellers risk being left out of the process.

Effects of Unsecured Land Tenure on Women's Contributions to Development

Secured land access (Adams 2004, p. 3) is a precondition for sustainable agriculture, poverty reduction and growth. This explains why countries with high Gin index (measure of national income inequality) are usually those with huge unequal distributions of landed property (World Bank 2003). Rural women particularly tend to favour sustainable environmental practices since by virtue of their reproductive roles they are responsible for water and firewood (Fonjong 2001; Negash 2006). With women having mere users' land rights, their ability to invest in land is reduced to basic seasonal short-term cultivation of food crops. The proceeds (cash and goods) thereof contribute to the education of children and the improvement of family welfare. These have the potential to uplift the standards of living and livelihood of households. But without security over land there is no guarantee that they will be able to continue assuming these roles. Women tend to farm on small plots and use land uniquely for seasonal food crops because of the uncertainty in their duration on the land. This has, for the most part, led to drops in yields and revenue. The result, as Goheen (1988) and Harms (1974) confirm, is that men own the land while women own the crops. This is a major source of domestic tension, given that women's over-dependence on men for land creates opportunities for potential gender-based conflicts when men attempt to control the proceeds that women derived from the land.

Unwritten customary laws encourage potential land conflicts in communities where shifting cultivation is still practised or where farming and grazing co-exist. These conflicts have been fuelled by the current competing demand and uses of land in the context of globalization. Be it the situation in Mali, Niger, Cote D'Ivoire, or Cameroon, where the problem has been heightened by other factors such as an increase in human and animal population, ecological and climate changes, and transhumance (Gefu & Kolawole 2002; Aredo 2005; Davidheiser & Luna 2008; Fonjong *et al.* 2010), unsecured land holding that stems from customary land instruments is at the root of the problem. Unfortunately, women usually end up paying the full price both during and after these conflicts in the form of crop destruction and displacement. In fact, 50 per cent of the women in this survey in Cameroon reported that they were forced to terminate farming activities in conflict areas in favour of the graziers and to resort to rented land, which increased their cost of production. The truth of the matter is that these women usually find themselves in weaker bargaining positions in the face of rich and powerful male cattle graziers who are able to buy justice from corrupt traditional and administrative authorities. This might be at the cost of food security for the entire community, but who really cares?

Conclusions

Patriarchy has constructed men as a class with power and dominance over women. The unequal power relation as a social construct is unethical and without any natural basis. It propels male economic and political agendas and privileges that are well packaged and delivered through customary practices in order to appeal to majority opinion in the society. Although these customs are not written, they are more powerful than written laws because they have been the norm over a long period of time. Despite the fact that they are abhorrent and discriminatory, they still pass for the living law by exploiting the weaknesses of statutory laws, which, even though gender neutral and non-discriminatory, cannot readily protect in practical terms the interests of women and other vulnerable groups.

Women, like men, are citizens and ought to share fundamental rights to natural resources, including land. Access to and ownership of land are issues of rights, survival and economic justice, and therefore gender discrimination should not continue, particularly in agrarian economies like Cameroon, given that those who have land command wealth and power. As such, discriminatory land practices only help to accentuate powerlessness among women and further the feminization of poverty. Unfortunately, the strong connectivity between land rights and the spirituality of the customary communities maintains the status quo, with low priority given to improving women's land rights in some developing societies.

Unlike the situation in the past, men are no longer the sole breadwinners of respective families and households. The number of single mothers is growing; the contribution of women to development at all levels is enormous. Customs which are both discriminatory and static are impediments to evolving societies and should no longer be given prominence in the present globalizing world. Good customs should advocate and promote the respect of human dignity and rights for all. Land reform is political and if customs in some poor countries are still far from meeting human rights objectives then governments need to act, as was the case in South Africa in 1994 and the Philippines in 1986, where changes in power led to better land reforms. Such gender-based reforms should be the outcome of broad-based consultation that is inclusive and addresses the questions of space, cost, procedure, and gender equality, bearing in mind that discrimination against women affects the whole of society. Improved women's access to, control and ownership of land/natural and productive resources, as Wandia (2009, p. 7) opines, are key factors in eradicating hunger and rural poverty.

There is, however, a glimmer of hope which needs to be sustained. Women in West Africa are gradually making claims over customary land, as seen among female rice producers in Ndop plain, Cameroon (Fonjong & Mbah 2007); low-lying rice swamps in Gambia; and Goin in south-western Burkina Faso. But the numbers of those involved and the pace of these changes are still areas of concern. The societal perception of women's ownership is also changing. The courts are assuming positive roles as bastions of justice and are ruling in favour of female inheritance. Though still timid, this is a positive departure from the strict orthodox tradition, which did not countenance female land inheritance or purchase. While Rao (2006, p. 181) cautions that this trend may not signify gender equality but points to a shift in the valuation of land and agriculture as livelihood resources and activities, land rights provide women with security and protection against violence and dispossession, increasing control over their sexuality and choices, and meeting their basic needs (Wandia 2009, p. 8). Women's land rights are thus no longer negotiable.

Acknowledgements

This study was carried out under Canadian International Development Research Centre (IDRC) Grant no. 105467 to the University of Buea. The authors gratefully acknowledge the comments, suggestions and editorial assistance of Cynthia Bisman in relation to the early drafts, which have impacted positively on this paper.

References

Adams, M. (2004) *Land Reform, Agriculture and Poverty Reduction*, working paper for the Renewable Natural Resources and Agriculture Team, Department for International Development (DFID) Policy Division, London, pp. 1–4.

Aluko, B. & Amidu, A. (2006) 'Women and Land Rights Reforms in Nigeria', paper presented at the 5th FIG regional conference on Promoting Land Administration and Good Governance, Accra, Ghana, 8–11 March.

Aredo, D. (2005) *Property Rights, Customary Institutions, and Conflict: The Case of the Southern Pastoral Areas of Ethiopia. Rural Common Property in a Perspective of Development and Modernization*, Addis Ababa University, Ethiopia.

Buchanan, I. & Gunn, R. (2007) 'The Interpretation of Human Rights in English Social Work: An Exploration in the Context of Services for Children and for Parents with Learning Difficulties', *Ethics and Social Welfare*, Vol. 1, no. 2, pp. 147–62.

Burnet, J. (n.d) *Women's Land Rights in Rwanda*, available at: <http://www.law.emory. edu/wandl/WAl-studies/rwanda.htm> (accessed 2 January 2012).

Cameroon Land Tenure Ordinance no. 74-I of 7 July 1974.

Cotula, L., Toulmin, C. & Hesse, C. (2004) *Land Tenure and Administration in Africa: Lessons of Experience and Emerging Issues*, International Institute for Environment and Development (IIED), London.

Davidheiser, M. & Luna, A.M. (2008) 'From Complementarity to Conflict: A Historical Analysis of Farmer-Fulbe Relations in West Africa', *African Journal on Conflict Resolution*, Vol. 8, no. 1, pp. 77–104.

Diaw, M.C. (1997) *Si, Nda bot and Ayong: Shifting Cultivation, Land Uses and Property Rights in Southern Cameroon*, ODI Rural Development Forestry Network, 21e, London, UK.

Ebi, J. (2008) 'The Structure of Succession Law in Cameroon: Finding a Balance between the Needs and Interests of Different Family Members', PhD thesis, University of Birmingham, UK.

Fissiy, C. (1992) *Power and Privilege in the Administration of Law*, African Studies Centre, Leiden.

Fonjong, L. (2001) 'Fostering Women's Participation in Development through Non-governmental Efforts in Cameroon', *Geographical Journal*, Vol. 167, no. 3, pp. 223–34.

Fonjong, L. & Mbah, F. (2007) 'The Fortunes and Misfortunes of Women Rice Producers in Ndop, Cameroon and the Implications for Gender Roles', *Journal of International Women's Studies*, Vol. 8, no. 4, pp. 133–47.

Fonjong, L., Sama-Lang, I. & Fombe, L. (2010) 'Assessment of the Evolution of Land Tenure System in Cameroon and its Effects on Women's Land Rights and Food Security', *Perspectives on Global Development and Technology (PGDT)*, Vol. 9, no. 1–2, pp. 154–69.

Friis, C. & Reenberg, A. (2010) *Land Grab in Africa: Emerging Land System Drivers in a Teleconnected World*, GLP Report no. 1, GLP International Project Office, University of Copenhagen.

Gefu, J.O. & Kolawole, A. (2002) 'Conflict in Common Property Resource Use: Experiences from an Irrigation Project'. Paper Prepared for 9th Conference of the International Association for the Study of Common Property, Indiana, available at: <http://d/c.dlib. Indiana.edu/achive/00000823/00/gefuj080502.pdf> (accessed 19 May 2009).

Goheen, M. (1988) 'Land and the Household Economy: Women Farmers of the Grassfields Today', in *Agriculture, Women and Land: The African Experience*, ed. J. Davison, Westview Press, Boulder, pp. 90–105.

Gray, L. & Kevane, M. (1999) 'Women and Land Tenure in Sub-Saharan Africa', *African Studies Review*, Vol. 42, no. 2, pp. 15–39.

Guivant, J. S. (2001) 'Gender and Land Rights in Brazil', paper prepared for the UNRISD Project on Agrarian Change, Gender and Land Rights, United Nations Research Institute for Social Development (UNRISD), Geneva.

Harms, R. (1974) *Land Tenure and Agricultural Development in Zaire, 1895–1961*, Land Tenure Center, Report no. 99, University of Wisconsin.

Kaberry, P. M. (1952) *Women of the Grass Fields*, HMSO, London.

Kambarami, M. (2006) *Culture, Feminity and Sexuality*, available at: <http://www.arsic. org/downloads/uhsss/kamabarami.pdf> (accessed 12 February 2010).

Karangathi, J. (2005) 'A Case Study on Common Property Tenure System (Kenya)', case study submitted for the joint study Rural Common Property in a Perspective of Development and Modernization, Mau Community Forest Association (MACOFA).

Lind, A. (2006) *Struggle and Development: Approaching Gender Bias in Practical International Development Work*, Orebro University, Orebro.

Moore, B. H. & Meinzen-Dick, R. (2008) 'Preface', in *Securing Common Property Regimes in a Globalizing World. Synthesis of 41 Case Studies on Common Property Regimes from Asia, Africa, Europe and Latin America*, by A. Fuys, E. Mwangi & S. Dohrn, International Land Coalition, Rome, p. v.

Mufeme, E. (1998) *Land: Breaking Bonds and Cementing Ties. Land and Spirituality in Africa*, available at: <http://www.wcc-coe.org/wcc/what/jpc/echoes-16-05.html> (accessed 14 September 2011).

Negash, A. (2006) *Economic Empowerment of Women*, available at: <http://www.scu. edu/ethics/practicing/focusareas/global_ethics/economicempowerment.html> (accessed February 2010).

Ngwafor, E. N. (1993) *Family Law in Anglophone Cameroon*, University of Regina Computer Services, Regina-Saskatchewan.

Njoh, A. (2002) 'Community and Change in Cameroonian Land Policy', *Planning Perspectives*, Vol. 15, no. 3, pp. 241–65.

Odhiambo, E. (2011) 'A Critique of the Land Reform Implementation Process in Kenya', National Stakeholders meeting on land reforms and decentralization organized by G10 Coalition, Panafric Hotel, Nairobi.

Palmer, R. (2002) *Gendered Land Rights—Process, Struggle, or Lost C(l)ause?*, Oxfam, Oxford.

Platteau, J. P., Abraham, A., Gaspart, F. & Stevens, L. (2005) 'Traditional Marriage Practices as Determinants of Women's Land Rights in Sub-Saharan Africa: A Review of Research', in *Gender and Land Compendium of Country Studies*, Food and Agricultural Organization, Rome, pp. 15–34.

Rao, N. (2006) 'Land Rights, Gender Equality and Household Food Security: Exploring the Conceptual Links in the Case of India', *Food Policy*, Vol. 31, no. 2, pp. 180–93.

Razavi, S. (2005) *Land Tenure Reform and Gender Equality*, UNRISD Policy Brief, UNRISD, Geneva, Switzerland, available at: <http://www.unrisd.org/80256B3C005BCCF9/http NetITFramePDF?> (accessed 12 July 2010).

Ribot, J. C. (2002) *African Decentralisation: Local Actors, Powers and Accountability*, UNRISD Programme on Democracy, Governance and Human Rights Paper no. 8, UNRISD, Geneva.

Rünger, M. (2006) 'Governance, Land Rights and Access to Land in Ghana—A Development Perspective on Gender Equity', paper presented at the 5th FIG regional conference on Promoting Land Administration and Good Governance, Accra, Ghana, 8–11 March.

United Nations Research Institute for Social Development (UNRISD) (2006) *Land Tenure Reform and Gender Equality*, UNRISD Research and Policy Brief no. 4, UNRISD, Geneva.

Wandia, M. (2009) 'Safeguarding Women's Rights Will Boost Food Security', *Pambazuka News*, 25 June, Issue 439, available at: <http://pambazuka.org/en/category/ features/57225>.

Whitehead, A. & Tsikata, D. (2003) 'Policy Discourses on Women's Land Rights in Sub-Saharan Africa: The Implications of the Return to the Customary', *Journal of Agrarian Change*, Vol. 3, no. 1 and 2, pp. 67–112.

Woodhouse, P. (2003) 'African Enclosures: A Default Mode of Development', *World Development*, Vol. 31, no. 1, pp. 1705–20.

World Bank (2003) 'Vice President's Foreword', in *Land Policies for Growth and Poverty Reduction*, by K. Deininger, World Bank, Washington, DC, pp. Xvii–lvi.

Gender Justice and Rights in Climate Change Adaptation: Opportunities and Pitfalls

Petra Tschakert and Mario Machado

We present three rights-based approaches to research and policies on gender justice and equity in the context of climate change adaptation. After a short introduction, we describe the dominant discourse that frames climate change and provide an overview of the literature that has depicted women both as vulnerable victims of climatic change and as active agents in adaptive responses. Discussion follows on the shift from gendered impacts to gendered adaptive capacities and embodied experiences, highlighting the continuing impact of social biases and institutional practices that shape unequal access to and control over household and community decision-making processes undermining timely, fair, and success-ful adaptive responses. Assessment of rights-based frameworks considers the space they provide in addressing persistent gender and other inequalities, at different political and operational scales. We argue that a human security framework is useful to fill the gap in current gender and climate justice work, particularly when implemented through the entry point of adaptive social protection. Gender justice in climate change adaptation is an obligation for transformational social change, not just rights. The time is ripe to replace narrow-minded vulnerability studies with a contextualized understanding of our mutual fragility and a commitment to enhanced livelihood resilience, worldwide.

Introduction

Dominant discourses on climate change adaptation have left little room for women to articulate their needs, rights, and responsibilities without being reduced to victims, a virtuous green consciousness, or responsible caretakers. In this paper, we examine research indicating that inequality with respect to gender as well as class, ethnicity, caste, etc. may undermine the potential of individuals, communities, and societies to be actively involved in and shape the transformative processes triggered by global environmental change. Undoubtedly, both men and women are impacted by droughts, floods, and heatwaves, and these impacts are experienced differently due to distinct roles determined by cultural norms, the gendered division of labor, and historically rooted practices and power structures. Such differential vulnerability is indicative of inequalities of power relations in any society.

We first introduce the dominant discourse on climate change adaptation and the various roles women play in adaptation narratives. Lessons from adaptation research illustrate that simplistic notions of women as vulnerable victims conceal deep-rooted inequalities, patterns of marginalization, and unequal power structures. To acknowledge these complexities and to progress forward, we then examine whether a rights-based approach could enrich current gender and climate change work by drawing attention to multiple and interconnected types of insecurities, and a contextualized understanding of both discriminatory mechanisms and our mutual fragility. Finally, we explore how rights perspectives may help to shift the climate change discourse from global managerialism to human relevance and immediacy, and from rights to empowerment and responsibilities. We propose a reframing of the rights discourse to one that stresses transformational change tightly linked to human security and justice as an obligation for change for all.

Climate Change Adaptation and the Role of Women

Global Managerialism

Climate change adaptation is typically understood as a responsive adjustment to the predicted impacts of future climate change. Rather than addressing the underlying processes that shape today's vulnerabilities, inequalities, and adaptive capacities—the ability to undertake adaptations or system changes—this dominant discourse assumes the function of bandaging the wound, not preventing this or future injuries from occurring. Embedded in such framing is the notion that people adapt through appropriate measures (typically technological in nature) and top-down policies and projects. The underlying premise is that stakeholders just need to choose the right adaptation strategy for a given locale and implement it. This assumes that the 'right' adaptation strategy is readily available, comprehensible and even possible, when in fact none of these may be true. Such a technocratic notion of adaptation is intrinsically linked to the concept of global managerialism (Adger *et al*. 2001). By reframing climate change from a social problem that is intractable to a technical problem, one succumbs to the illusion of having control, rather than accepting the complexity and unpredictability of social behavior and the messiness of political decision making.

Such a reductionist perspective of climate change as a scientific and technological problem is an inherently flawed approach to a 'wicked problem', one that is difficult or impossible to solve because of its complex and changing interdependencies. Feminist researchers have critiqued it as the ultimate form of hegemonic masculinity (e.g. Alaimo 2009; Seager 2009; MacGregor 2010). Alaimo (2009), for instance, argues that predominant notions of neutrality (both scientific and political) in climate change science not only avoid explicit language of risk, danger, and harm but also purposefully obscure underlying uncertainties, as an excuse for apathy. Likewise, MacGregor (2010) cautions that 'masculine risk-taking and the quest of progress' (p. 133), exemplified in complex technologies and innovations in mitigation and adaptation policies (e.g. carbon trading and genetically modified crops), favor the new and progressive rather than the old and well served. Therefore, the managerial discourse renders invisible local experiences with climatic variability, agency, and autonomous adaptive strategies of the most vulnerable.

Women as Vulnerable Victims

Whereas women's role in the global scientific discourses and policy debates on climate change has remained partial and largely silenced, women have featured prominently in the adaptation debate, yet mainly as vulnerable victims, particularly in the Global South. Time and again feminist authors have critiqued this biased perspective that perpetuates negative stereotypes of a Southern woman as 'helpless, voiceless and largely unable to manage herself'. Similarly Resurreccion (2011) critiques the portrayal of women as 'chief victim-and-caretaker': despite their presumably inherent vulnerability, women often act as crucial agents in adaptation programs. Such uncritical emphasis on women's knowledge, roles, and responsibilities, without an explicit consideration of power analysis, is likely to exacerbate the 'feminization of responsibility' (Arora-Jonsson 2011).

It could be argued that this vulnerabilization of women, especially poor women, helps policy debates to put gender aspects and unequal gender relations on the map. Yet giving way to such pressures, simplifying complex power structures, and sloganizing narratives reinforce gender myths and promote misleading feminist fables (Cornwall *et al.* 2007). Moreover, an overemphasis on women's universal vulnerability not only denies women agency, knowledge, and resilience and positions their vulnerability as their intrinsic problem, it also masks power imbalances and prevents the confrontation of something concrete and factual (Arora-Jonsson 2011). Most importantly, such framing obfuscates the drivers that put women in such precarious conditions, in other words *who* and *what* makes them vulnerable (Cuomo 2011).

An additional danger in such one-sided representations lies in the portrayal of women's roles as static, ignoring how vulnerability is produced and reproduced in daily life. Yet gender roles, obligations, and tasks in climate change adaptation are rarely fixed, but instead are negotiated and contested as a reflection of new constraints and emerging opportunities that operate within the dynamic context of daily life. Moreover, cultural norms can also cause enhanced gender-specific vulnerability among men, such as male risk taking (machismo) under Hurricane Mitch in Nicaragua and the attempts of primarily young West African men to enter Europe through the dangerous boat route, both of which have caused high numbers of male deaths (Bradshaw 2010).

Women as Agents of Change

More recent work directs attention to gendered agency, skills, voices, and experiences with past extreme weather events and climatic variability. This trend not only attempts to correct the 'troubling binary between universal (scientific) masculine knowledge and the marked vulnerability of impoverished women' (Alaimo 2009, p. 30) but also contests the uncritical acceptance of the scientific framing of climate change in general, and the long prevailing impacts-focus in climate change adaptation in particular. Methodologically, this means moving away from descriptive vulnerability assessments to diagnosing drivers of inequality, marginalization, and barriers to transformative change, and promoting agency and resilience through processes of engagement and collective learning.

While recent counter-narratives have successfully avoided positioning women, especially those in the Global South, as inherent victims of climate change and perpetuating gender differences, caution is still required not to go overboard to the other extreme. The notion of feminization of (environmental) responsibility also holds true for women in the North. An overemphasis on women's 'virtue' in climate change (Arora-Jonsson 2011) is equally simplistic. Not only does it present women in the North as a homogeneous entity, again concealing inequalities in decision making, but it also transfers responsibility to individual women in their homes, fulfilling their green consumerism gender roles, rather than addressing the climate challenge at the level of governments and industries. Such a framing risks further entrenching social gender roles and perpetuating inequalities.

Gendered Adaptive Capacities and Embodied Experiences

The most recent debates on gender and climate change reflect two schools of thought: one is rooted in critical adaptation work that illustrates why climate impacts are gendered (rather than just diagnosing impacts) and why social differentiation is crucial for evaluating the very processes and conditions that perpetuate gender inequalities and those that enhance adaptive capacities; the other, taking a feminist poststructural lens, sees vulnerability as an embodied experience that transcends disconnected identities across space and time.

Adaptive capacity—the ability to undertake adaptive measures—is shaped by a set of determinants, including perceptions, access to communication networks, insurance, and credit, and risk-sharing mechanisms. For some, this shift from impacts to capacities lies at the heart of 'climate justice' debates. It focuses explicitly on gender division of labor, labor mobility, and decision-making structures, at the level of households and communities, as intrinsically and dynamically shaped by social and cultural norms. Such a focus pays close attention to social biases and differentiation that risk impeding rather than enhancing adaptive capacities, as well as discriminatory institutional practices that undermine timely, fair, and successful adaptive responses. An adaptive capacity lens is also sensitive to gender-specific vulnerabilities of men, linked to poverty or limited access to resources, cultural expectations, and vulnerabilities that stem from inequalities due to class, age, ethnicity, and caste.

Recent case studies have demonstrated the different roles that women and men take on in both the Global North and South that cause differential impacts and responses. For instance, Alston (2011), in her work on climate change and a 10-year drought in rural Australia, found that men faced higher suicide levels resulting from the tasks carried out as a response to the drought (e.g. destroying frail animals) and the social isolation, loss of political power, and attacks on male identity and masculinity that surround loss in rurality. By contrast, women took on off-farm work, resulting in more interaction at the community level, in addition to assisting with on-farm tasks and caring for their families' and neighbors' health, often at the expense of their own.

Cases from adaptation projects in Vietnam (Oxfam and United Nations Vietnam 2009) confirm such gendered vulnerabilities and adaptive responses. For instance, gender allocation of household food supplies during periods of prolonged food shortages favors men while women suffer from a lower caloric intake. Health impacts, especially waterborne diseases, affect women and children disproportionally. Violence against women after disasters increases while mortality among men due to search and rescue efforts seems higher. Workloads often rise for both men and women, although differently in type and timing, contingent on gender norms that influence social behavior. A study from Cambodia (Resurreccion 2011) further underscores the highly dynamic adaptation strategies that both men and women undertake in response to altered cropping cycles. These include men logging trees and engaging in charcoal production for sale, despite cultural taboos, while women engage in wage labor and raising livestock at home.

For other researchers, especially feminist materialist theorists, this evolution in discourse and practice fails to reach far enough, despite considerable improvement compared to the early impact studies. The argument is that a focus on adaptive capacity nevertheless restricts the main emphasis on autonomous individuals treated as concrete measurable beings while ignoring embodied experiences that transcend locales and dynamic, fragmented identities (Elmhirst 2011). By building on what Alaimo (2009, p. 23) calls 'trans-corporeality', this strand of literature zooms in on embodied connections and experiences as a relationship to others, including those that inhibit the over-consuming world, the global inequalities it perpetuates, and the science framings and knowledge regimes that monitor, quantify, and govern the vulnerable.

What Can a Rights-based Approach Add to the Gender and Adaptation Debate?

Insights from climate change adaptation research and feminist theory demon-strate that without addressing and rectifying practices that perpetuate social biases and discriminatory attitudes and structures, gender inequalities and associated gendered vulnerabilities and adaptive capacities are unlikely to change. This requires a shift in perspective, from needs to rights. Researchers in development ethics and feminist science have argued for a rights-based approach (RBA) as a practical lens through which to assess climate change without necessarily pointing fingers over past and future emissions and historic respon-sibilities. It offers relational narratives that humanize the complexity of the problem, incorporating fairness and responsibilities, while also providing room for engagement rather than just descriptive analysis. This constitutes a discursive re-construction of climate change, from an economic and technological framing to a social framing. It asks what climate change means to you, to me, and to other people in different parts of the world. Presumably, this lens allows us to unmask pre-existing inequalities, disempowerment, chronic poverty, and structural violence, all of which inhibit successful and just adaptation to climatic and other stressors and shocks. We review three entry points to a RBA and identify opportunities and possible pitfalls for gender and climate change adaptation.

Human Rights and Climate Change: The Legal Dimension

In March 2008, the United Nations Human Rights Council adopted Resolution 7/23 on human rights and climate change. It explicitly recognized that climate change 'has implications for the full enjoyment of human rights' (UNHRC, preamble). A petition filed by the Inuit of Canada and the United States in 2005 and the 2007 Malé Declaration from the Maldives first stipulated that climate change represented a violation of human rights of the poor and of future generations. As a consequence, the Office of the High Commissioner for Human Rights in an unprecedented study reports that the impacts of climate change directly implicate specific rights including the right to life, the right to adequate food, the right to water, the right to health, the right to adequate housing, and the right to self-determination (OHCHR 2009, pp. 21–41).

Adopting a human rights lens at the state level is likely to take time. We suspect that it may not consider gender and gender inequalities as high priorities.

While a RBA can create individual imperatives to act and amplify the voices of those who are disproportionally affected, there are theoretical and practical barriers to the adoption of such a framework. Limon (2009) argues that an explicit focus on the right to a safe and secure environment may be most effective as an extension to environmental rights that permit quality of life, dignity, and well-being.

A Rights-based Approach to Development and Human Capabilities

Research on gender and adaptation has much to learn from development rights, development ethics, and global ethics. Shue (1980) laid out the cornerstones for economic human rights, including the basic right to subsistence or minimum economic security, meaning 'unpolluted air, unpolluted water, adequate food, adequate clothing, adequate shelter, and minimal preventive public health care' (p. 23). He introduced correlative duties that, beyond being simply 'positive' and 'negative' rights (dos and don'ts), consist of duties to avoid depriving, duties to protect from deprivation, and duties to aid the deprived. Most relevant is his reasoning on the allocation of duty and responsibility as his principle of priority for vital interests.

Equally relevant for justice under climate change are the contributions to development ethics from Sen (1985, 1999) and Nussbaum (2001) regarding human functioning, capabilities, and flourishing. While Sen put agency at the center of his analysis on rights to freedom, Nussbaum emphasized control over one's political environment as a means for citizen participation. Although the capabilities approach continues to be influential, particularly among policy makers and development experts, it has failed to produce useful practical applications, including empowering methodologies (Robeyns 2006).

In development studies, RBAs pinpoint structural causes of poverty and inequality, identify material and political constraints and unequal power relations that prevent the securing of rights, and open spaces for participation and good governance. They can secure structural change and protect the poor, with rights-bearing actors and duty bearers at their core (Hickey & Mitlin 2009). Such a relational claim is directly relevant to vulnerable people with rights not just needs, with knowledge, skills, and agency not just passive survival strategies.

Examples from adaptation projects suggest that focusing on gendered entitlements (different types of assets or capitals) and gendered capabilities is most useful for addressing persistent gender inequalities. For instance, Oxfam and United Nations Vietnam (2009) identified specific gender and power dynamics in rural Vietnam—participation in household decision making, involvement in community social activities, and participation in local political and management structures—as key determinants of how effectively men and women were able to mediate climate change impacts. Lacking agency often translated into lower resilience during disasters. While such lessons confirm that adaptive capacity is differentiated along gender and social lines, they have little to offer to enforce duties and responsibilities and correct the very dynamics that propagate injustices.

Global Ethics and Human Security

So far, we have argued that the most significant gaps in research on gender and climate change adaptation concern the difficulty in addressing and remedying the social biases and discriminatory institutional practices that create unequal access to and control over household and community decision making and restrict adaptive capacities. They, in turn, undermine timely, fair, and successful adaptive responses. We now propose a conceptual and practical approach that tackles persistent gender inequalities, from the perspective of climate change as an intrinsically social challenge.

We first draw upon global ethics to delineate the broader frame. McNeill and St. Clair (2011) argue that global ethics and global justice, particularly through the works of Pogge (2007, 2010) and Young (2004), have re-introduced the concept of responsibility into fighting poverty and structural injustice. While Pogge favors a global institutional order to eliminate poverty, Young underscores the obligation of moral agents, both individual and collective, as fundamentally shaped by social relations. Hence, it is this response-ability for participating in, and potentially benefiting from, social structures that expose others to harm that functions as an obligation for justice (McNeill & St. Clair 2011). This demarcates global ethics as arguably the most prominent rights framework of relevance to the challenges posed by climate change.

Gasper (2010) and O'Brien *et al.* (2010) propose human security as a framework that complements and enriches the language of rights and develop-ment as discussed within global ethics. The human security framework, distinct from an environmental (and national) security approach, is uniquely positioned to confront complex issues such as climate change as well as social inequalities, including gender inequalities, as it represents a synthesis of key ideas from human development, human rights, capabilities, and the basic needs discourses. It refers to the security of 'basic needs life-areas' (Gasper 2010) and, hence, constitutes an implicit basic rights claim. Human security is distinctly people centered, with an explicit emphasis on people's options to confront threats to their rights and the capacity and freedom to exercise these options (GECHS 1999). Despite concerns about the 'securitization' of the concept, it holds the potential for an integrated agenda of social justice, gender and race equality, and an ethical and emancipatory lens that focuses on those most in need, and the protection of essential environmental resources and services, locally and globally (Matthew *et al.* 2009). Recent attempts by feminist scholars employing a human security framework to address gendered vulnerabilities in global/climate change (e.g. Goldsworthy 2010; MacGregor 2010; Resurreccion 2011), we argue, fail to highlight persistent inequalities on multiple fronts.

First, a human security lens engages directly with notions of rights and responsibilities, and the recognition of the obligations associated with them (Anand & Gasper 2007). It expands the individualistic notion of capabilities, self-fulfillment, and the right to self-determination to an inclusive commitment to the well-being of others. Moreover, it provides the necessary ethical space to embrace holistic and global notions of sympathy, interconnectedness, and recognition of our mutual fragility. It aims to connect with the lives of *real* people, understanding development as a collective social process in which everyone holds a vested interest.

Second, it promotes empowerment among citizens, poor and rich in both developed and developing countries, not just rights. The geographic span dismantles the old North–South dichotomy in which the (rich) Global North provides aid and the (poor) Global South accepts with indebtedness. Highlighting individual empowerment, embedded in felt experiences and shared security, means facilitating changes in consciousness and daily decision making (Kabeer 2011). Thus, a human security lens puts transformation at the core of its analysis.

Third, it includes the responsibility to protect those who are less fortunate, built into a reflexive process that questions how progress is defined and on whose expense it is pursued (St. Clair 2010). It also reflects bearing witness to those subject to structural violence, through compassion, a culture of solidarity, and activism, as well as the cultivation of moral responsibility and responsible caring attitudes and actions as advocated in feminist ethics of care (Cuomo 2011).

Fourth, it provides an ethically defendable counterweight to the seemingly just cost–benefit analyses that dominate the economics-driven assessments in climate change research. Instead of favoring monetary value and highest purchasing power, which mask deep-rooted gender, class, caste, ethnic, and intergenerational injustices (Gasper 2010), human security recognizes the equal worth of people. This framing mirrors Nelson's call for an 'ethically transparent, real-world-oriented, and flexible economic practice' (2008, p. 441). Quantifiable 'objective' science results, while commendable for their ease of understanding, belie the true complexity of the human condition to the detriment of those most desperately in need of development.

Finally, human security challenges underlying neo-liberal thinking that promotes the personhood and social fragmentation rather than solidarity, social citizenship, and obligations to and for others (Gledhill 2009). It provides a means to increase resilience for people, especially important after economic recession and neo-liberal cutbacks on social services when old 'safety nets' have been eroded and no new economic opportunities arise under market-driven policies. Neo-liberalism, according to Harvey (2005), achieves only the dehumanization of social problems, by reducing the moral imperative of society to the preservation of individual freedom and by labeling free enterprise (the free market) as the ultimate expression of its mantra.

Adaptive Social Protection and Social Work

Operationalizing global ethics and human security under climate change is an enormous challenge, particularly as it involves eradicating persistent gender and other inequalities that undermine adaptive capacity and successful adaptation. We see most potential through adaptive social protection (ASP). The concept of ASP merges community-based adaptation with proactive disaster risk management and social protection. It aims to build resilience among the poor and disenfranchised by countering intrinsic vulnerability, addressing unsafe living conditions, and boosting people's ability to reduce risks and promote livelihood transformations (Arnall *et al.* 2010). Transformative measures attempt to empower people to exercise their voice, combat discrimination, claim the right to protection when state or private safety nets fail, and transform social relations. This includes rectifying gendered inequalities in entitlements and capabilities often perpetuated through gendered social norms and division of labor.

Several projects (e.g. Oxfam, CARE International, Practical Action) have emerged that adopt ASP as a practical implementation of a human security framework, some focused specifically on gender dimensions. For instance, a community-based adaptation project in Nepal allows for critical unpacking of gender norms in farming practices that determine adaptive responses to climatic stress. Rarer are transformative projects such as one in Bangladesh that promotes skills training among poor, vulnerable, and socially excluded women to transform livelihoods, rather than boosting coping strategies, thereby explicitly ousting encrusted layers of inequality (Arnall *et al.* 2010). These examples evoke a notable shift from conventional food-for-work programs to dynamic support structures that target predictable and recurrent needs under climatic uncertainty.

Nonetheless, not all programs tackle gender inequalities at their roots. In Senegal, socially marginalized women have become mitigators of climate change on their own terms through reforestation and energy management programs (WEDO 2008). They contribute to their own livelihood security (e.g. increasing availability of fuel-wood, generating financial resources) while establishing their roles as community leaders. Although these women embody the role of agents for change, outcomes mirror the above-discussed 'feminization of responsibility' rather than structural changes in power relations. The danger is that such low yardsticks in gender empowerment become the norm and, subsequently, are mainstreamed into governmental policies while forsaking true empowerment and flourishing outside of pre-defined gender roles.

Similarly, reports on adaptive responses to the 2007 massive rainfall in Ghana suggest, at first glance, that women were able to diversify their livelihoods through alternative cash crops (WEDO 2008). However, Carr (2008) shows how adaptive measures mobilize existing gender roles and power relations in production, consistently to the detriment of women. Ghana's Livelihood Empowerment Against Poverty (LEAP) program, employing smartcards, mobile ATMs, and cell phones for immediate cash transfers (Ellis *et al.* 2009), may provide the right stimulus for women, elderly people, and caregivers to break out of this vicious cycle.

So far, pilots of these climate- and disaster-focused adaptive social protection programs exist in developing countries only. While cynics may argue that they represent nothing more than old development projects in new disguises, we assert that there is an enormous potential also to implement ASP in the Global North, merging its key tenets with existing social work and social welfare policies. First attempts to link social work and environmental issues are emerging, although clear gender dimensions are yet to be articulated. Norton (2011), for instance, examines how social work and ecosystem sustainability are linked through empathy and empowerment, drawing parallels between the oppression of women and domination of nature. Dominelli (2011) and Peeters (2012) encourage active participation of social workers in raising community awareness about climate change, challenging the social, political, and economic structures behind the climate problem and persistent structural inequalities. Bell (2012) advocates for interconnectedness, wholeness, diversity, embodiment, situated knowledge, and inclusiveness that support the human rights foundation of social work. Her emphasis is on relationships in social work and the processes that generate knowledge on embodied experiences and restore and enact 'epistemic agency to disempowered people' (p. 419).

While not focused on climate change per se, we argue that Bell's framework sets the stage for using a human security lens in action. This is particularly urgent as poverty in medium- and high-income countries is on the rise. Stressing poor people's agency and resilience rather than powerlessness and material deprivation is critical. Yet more attention is needed to understand how social protection has worked for the poor in welfare states (e.g. Scandinavia) compared to welfare programs squeezed by neo-liberal policies in which the poor are constructed as a category outside all responsible social relations (Lawson & St. Clair 2009), witnessed in New Orleans after Hurricane Katrina.

Discussion and Conclusion

In light of the various rights-based frameworks presented here and their respective merit for gender justice in climate change adaptation, we argue that the most pressing need is an explicit focus on positive change that goes beyond narrow definitions of rights. While such change often stems from legal discourses and practices about rights, transformational change goes deeper, challenging the ways in which subjects (women, men, the poor, etc.) are produced and re-produced and act in relation to the exercise of power across the globe. A human security lens, implemented through adaptive social protection programs, brings the idea of 'security' full circle by demonstrating that true 'security' cannot be a product of isolationism. By revisiting the meaning of personal security overlaid by a dialogue of interconnectedness and mutual fragility, human security becomes a transformative framework that works against deep-seated power structures that inhibit the security of all people.

The conventional world dichotomy across North—South lines dissolves once we see vulnerability as an embodied experience felt by each and every single human being; vulnerability as a shared (albeit unequal) experience becomes the impetus for change, from the smallest level (the body) to international relations.

We capture this interconnectedness by showing the interlinked scales, both spatial and temporal, at which human security emerges and transforms social relations (see Figure 1). We stress two aspects: (1) expressions of threats and opportunities apply to both highly industrialized nations and least-developed countries; and (2) gender is all but one subjectivity counted under 'intersectionality', the intersection of gender, race, ethnicity, sexuality, etc. (Nightingale 2011). Gender inequalities and vulnerabilities often occur in concert with other inequalities and vulnerabilities, resulting in synergistic and reinforcing constraints. Gender is one element of the multiple and fragmented identities that one individual may inhabit that shapes or hinders successful adaptive responses under climate change. A human security lens suspends discrete scales by viewing connectedness as a continuum, ranging from localized daily experiences to a global ethics of care.

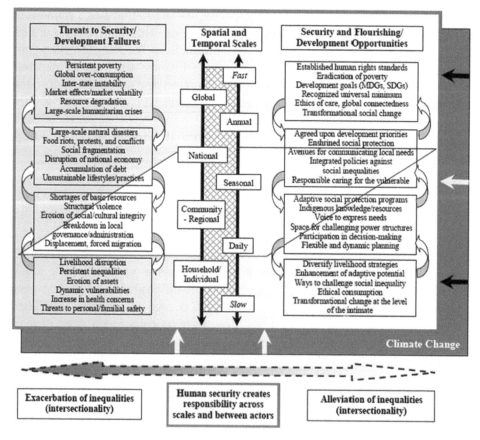

Figure 1. Understanding human security across dynamic spatial and temporal scales, with climate change as an additional layer of complexity.

We understand gender justice as an obligation for change, not just rights. This counterbalances the drawbacks associated with a narrow rights framework that often defies responsibilities to other people and to nature, as well as the responsibility to hold accountable institutions of social well-being. Local and international NGOs may also be reluctant to adopt a RBA in that non-compliable rights-holders and duty-bearers could exacerbate unequal power relations. Also RBA is often driven by external legal experts and rights movements who confront the state and other duty-bearers, irrespective of the potentially even more contentious relations left behind. In climate change, innovative autonomous adaptation highlights local adaptive capacity through experimentation and self-organization, in the absence of pro-poor national adaptation plans, though limits to self-help should be identified and flagged.

Undoubtedly, more work is needed to explore in depth the gender dimensions and pitfalls of emerging adaptive social protection programs. While we see a concrete opening through which to implement a human security approach that is sensitive to gender concerns and lingering inequalities in adaptation programs, no convincing evidence exists yet that illustrates how to link the self-interests of people and states across the globe. We simply lack a functional prototype that allows us to engage in true connectedness and shared embodied experiences throughout our socially fragmented world.

How do we *do* human security? In addition to social protection programs, we argue for the incorporation of a 'universal social minimum' (Davies *et al.* 2009) into climate negotiations. What we need is a model of deliberate democracy in which ethically motivated individuals, corporations, and governments act on their caring and initiate wide-ranging structural transformation. Affluent institutions may pay a base premium for poor and socially excluded people to participate in index-based weather insurance programs, or support other social services that boost adaptive capacity. Private equity offsets that facilitate emission-reducing behavior at home can support equity-enhancing and emission-reduction projects abroad. From a research and practitioners' perspective, we endorse a conduct of caring and immediacy that promotes agency, livelihood and ecosystem resilience, and transformational change through processes of engagement and collective learning. The time is ripe to replace vulnerability studies with inequality assessments that scrutinize the social, economic, political, and cultural drivers that perpetuate discrimination and injustices. The era that permitted perpetrators to renege on their human responsibilities by retreating under the cloak of personal freedom is over.

References

Adger, W. N., Benjaminsen, T. A., Brown, K. & Svarstad, H. (2001) 'Advancing a Political Ecology of Global Environmental Discourses', *Development and Change*, Vol. 32, no. 4, pp. 681–715.

Alaimo, S. (2009) 'Insurgent Vulnerability and the Carbon Footprint of Gender', *Kvinder, Køn & Forskning*, Vol. 3, pp. 22–35.

Alston, M. (2011) 'Gender and Climate Change in Australia', *Journal of Sociology*, Vol. 47, no. 1, pp. 53–70.

Anand, P. B. & Gasper, D. (2007) 'Guest Editorial: Conceptual Framework and Overview. Special Issue on Human Security, Well-being and Sustainability: Rights, Responsibilities and Priorities', *Journal of International Development*, Vol. 19, no. 4, pp. 449–56.

Arnall, A., Oswald, K., Davies, M., Mitchell, T. & Coirolo, C. (2010) *Adaptive Social Protection: Mapping the Evidence and Policy Context in the Agriculture Sector in South Asia*, IDS Working Paper 345, Institute of Development Studies, Brighton.

Arora-Jonsson, S. (2011) 'Virtue and Vulnerability: Discourses on Women, Gender and Climate Change', *Global Environmental Change*, Vol. 21, no. 2, pp. 744–51.

Bell, K. (2012) 'Towards a Post-conventional Philosophical Base for Social Work', *British Journal of Social Work*, Vol. 42, no. 3, pp. 408–23.

Bradshaw, S. (2010) 'Women, Poverty, and Disasters: Exploring the Links through Hurricane Mitch in Nicaragua', in *International Handbook of Gender and Poverty*, ed. S. Chant, Edward Elgar, Cheltenham, pp. 627–32.

Carr, E. (2008) 'Between Structure and Agency: Livelihoods and Adaptation in Ghana's Central Region', *Global Environmental Change*, Vol. 18, no. 4, pp. 689–99.

Cornwall, A., Harrison, E. & Whitehead, A. (2007) 'Gender Myths and Feminist Fables: The Struggle for Interpretive Power in Gender and Development', *Development and Change*, Vol. 38, no. 1, pp. 1–20.

Cuomo, C. (2011) 'Climate Change, Vulnerability, and Responsibility', *Hypatia*, Vol. 26, no. 4, pp. 690–714.

Davies, M., Oswald, K. & Mitchell, T. (2009) 'Climate Change Adaptation, Disaster Risk Reduction and Social Protection', in *Promoting Pro-poor Growth: Social Protection*, OECD, Paris, pp. 201–17.

Dominelli, L. (2011) 'Climate Change: Social Workers' Roles and Contributions to Policy Debates and Interventions', *International Journal of Social Welfare*, Vol. 20, no. 4, pp. 430–8.

Ellis, F., Devereux, S. & White, P. (2009) *Social Protection in Africa*, Edward Elgar, Cheltenham, UK and Northampton, MA.

Elmhirst, R. (2011) 'Introducing New Feminist Political Ecologies', *Geoforum*, Vol. 42, no. 2, pp. 129–32.

Gasper, D. (2010) *Climate Change and the Language of Human Security*, ISS Working Papers—General Series no. 505, ISS, The Hague, pp. 1–28.

GECHS (1999) *Science Plan: Global Environmental Change and Human Security*, International Human Dimensions Programme, Bonn.

Gledhill, J. (2009) 'The Rights of the Rich versus the Rights of the Poor', in *Rights-based Approaches to Development: Exploring the Potential and Pitfalls*, eds S. Hickey & D. Mitlin, Kumarian Press, Sterling, VA, pp. 31–48.

Goldsworthy, H. (2010) 'Women, Global Environmental Change, and Human Security', in *Global Environmental Change and Human Security*, eds R. A. Matthew, J. Barnett, B. McDonald & K. O'Brien, MIT Press, Cambridge, MA and London, pp. 215–36.

Harvey, D. (2005) *A Brief History of Neoliberalism*, Oxford University Press, New York.

Hickey, S. & Mitlin, D. (2009) 'Introduction', in *Rights-based Approaches to Development: Exploring the Potential and Pitfalls*, eds S. Hickey & D. Mitlin, Kumarian Press, Sterling, VA, pp. 3–20.

Kabeer, N. (2011) Empowerment, Citizenship and Gender Justice: A Contribution to Locally-grounded Theories of Social Change, plenary talk at the 9th international conference of the International Development Ethics Association: 'Gender Justice and Development: Global and Local', Bryn Mawr, PA, 9–11 June.

Lawson, V. & St. Clair, A. L. (2009) 'Global Poverty Studies and Human Security', *IHDP Update*, Vol. 2, pp. 35–9.

Limon, M. (2009) 'Human Rights and Climate Change: Constructing a Case for Political Action', *Harvard Environmental Law Review*, Vol. 33, no. 2, pp. 439–76.

MacGregor, S. (2010) 'A Stranger Silence Still: The Need for Feminist Social Research on Climate Change', *Sociological Review*, Vol. 57, no. 3, pp. 124–40.

Matthew, R. A., Barnett, J., McDonald, B. & O'Brien, K. L. (2009) *Global Environmental Change and Human Security*, MIT Press, Cambridge, MA.

McNeill, D. & St. Clair, A. L. (2011) 'Poverty, Human Rights, and Global Justice: The Response-ability of Multilateral Organizations', *Globalizations*, Vol. 8, no. 1, pp. 97–111.

Nelson, J. (2008) 'Economists, Value Judgments, and Climate Change: A View from Feminist Economics', *Ecological Economics*, Vol. 65, no. 3, pp. 441–7.

Nightingale, A. (2011) 'Bounding Difference: Intersectionality and the Material Production of Gender, Caste, Class, and Environment in Nepal', *Geoforum*, Vol. 42, no. 2, pp. 153–62.

Norton, C. L. (2011) 'Social Work and the Environment: An Ecosocial Approach', *International Journal of Social Welfare*, DOI: 10.1111/j.1468-2397.2011.00853.x

Nussbaum, M. (2001) *Women and Human Development: The Capabilities Approach*, Cambridge University Press, Cambridge.

O'Brien, K., St. Clair, A. L. & Kristoffersen, B. (eds) (2010) *Climate Change, Ethics, and Human Security*, Cambridge University Press, Cambridge.

Office of the UN High Commissioner for Human Rights (OHCHR) (2009) *Report of the Office of the UN High Commissioner for Human Rights on the Relationship Between Human Rights and Climate Change*, UN Doc. A/HRC/10/61 [15 Jan 2009].

Oxfam and United Nations Vietnam (2009) *Responding to Climate Change in Viet Nam: Opportunities for Improving Gender Equality. A Policy Discussion Paper*, Oxfam and United Nations Vietnam, Ha Noi.

Peeters, J. (2012) 'A Comment on "Climate Change: Social Workers' Roles and Contributions to Policy Debates and Interventions"', *International Journal of Social Welfare*, Vol. 21, no. 1, pp. 105–7.

Pogge, T. (ed.) (2007) *Freedom from Poverty as a Human Right: Who Owes What to the Very Poor*, Oxford University Press, Oxford.

Pogge, T. (2010) *Politics as Usual: What Lies behind the Pro-poor Rhetoric*, Polity Press, London.

Resurreccion, B. (2011) *The Gender and Climate Change Debate: More of the Same or New Pathways of Thinking and Doing?*, Asia Security Initiative Policy Series Working Paper no. 10, RSIS Centre for Non-traditional Security Studies, Singapore.

Robeyns, I. (2006) 'The Capability Approach in Practice', *Journal of Political Philosophy*, Vol. 14, no. 3, pp. 351–76.

Seager, J. (2009) 'Death by Degrees: Taking a Feminist Hard Look at the 2° Climate Policy', *Kvinder, Køn & Forskning*, Vol. 3, pp. 11–21.

Sen, A. (1985) 'Well-being, Agency and Freedom: The Dewey Lectures 1984', *Journal of Philosophy*, Vol. 82, no. 4, pp. 169–221.

Sen, A. (1999) *Development as Freedom*, Alfred A. Knopf, New York.

Shue, H. (1980) *Basic Rights: Subsistence, Affluence, and U.S. Foreign Policy*, Princeton University Press, Princeton.

St. Clair, A. (2010) 'Global Poverty and Climate Change: Towards the Responsibility to Protect', in *Climate Change, Ethics and Human Security*, eds K. O'Brien, A. St. Clair & B. Kristoffersen, Cambridge University Press, Cambridge, pp. 180–98.

Women's Environment and Development Organization (WEDO) (2008) *Gender, Climate Change and Human Security: Lessons from Bangladesh, Ghana, and Senegal*, WEDO, New York, pp. 1–73.

Young, I. (2004) 'Responsibility and Global Labor Justice', *Journal of Political Philosophy*, Vol. 12, no. 4, pp. 365–88.

Integrating Peace, Justice and Development in a Relational Approach to Peacebuilding

Jennifer J. Llewellyn

This paper considers how restorative justice as a theory of justice grounded in feminist relational theory can offer a conceptual framework from which to understand and approach justice, peace and development and their interrelationship in the context of peacebuilding. Feminist relational theory grounds a conception of justice that moves beyond the narrow focus on justice as merely an element or stage of peacebuilding to an understanding of peacebuilding as the work of building sustainable just social relationships.

Introduction: The Dilemmas in Current Accounts of Peacebuilding

In his report *In Larger Freedom* Secretary General Kofi Annan prefaced his proposal for the creation of a UN Peacebuilding Commission with the alarming estimate that '[r]oughly half of all countries that emerge from war lapse back into violence within five years' (Annan 2005, chap. 3, para. 114). He identified 'a gaping hole in the UN institutional machinery: no part of the UN system effectively addresses the challenges of helping countries with the transition from war to lasting peace' (chap. 3, para. 114). This telling failure suggests that for peace to be sustainable it cannot simply be *made* through security and/or justice interventions; it must, instead, be *built* through multi-pronged and integrated strategies. This insight underlies the logic of the UN Peacebuilding

Commission's focus on coordination and integration of these activities in order to achieve lasting results.

The Peacebuilding Commission's approach to this issue has, however, been primarily operational. The mandate of the Commission is to assist, enable and empower post-conflict states to develop and bring to fruition their own vision for peace and the path to achieving it. This approach clearly reflects a commitment to contextualized strategies that recognize and respond to the particularities of the society in question. The Commission's means of achieving this work has been to bring together the actors and agencies responsible for these activities and interventions and encourage them to share information with one another and coordinate their efforts largely through meetings and a common reporting structure. But five years after its advent, the mandated review of the Commission concluded that these efforts have been disappointing at best (United Nations 2010, Executive Summary).

Some have advocated sequencing as the appropriate strategy to resolve tensions in the demands of peacebuilding.[1] But while coordination and complementarity are valuable, I argue, new policies and institutions alone are inadequate. This view was shared by the review committee for the Peacebuilding Commission that acknowledged the 'illusion of sequencing':

> There is acceptance in all quarters that sequencing does not work, that effective peacebuilding must not follow peacekeeping operations but accompany them from their inception... Despite this acknowledgement, there is a widespread sense that the sequential approach remains the dominant one at the United Nations. Even if modest elements of peacebuilding are incorporated in mandates, the focus and mindset of operations is a peacekeeping one. Peacebuilding tends to be viewed as an add-on during the lifetime of the peacekeeping operation, expected to come into its own in the aftermath. Such a sequential approach neither gives adequate weight to peacebuilding nor responds to needs and realities on the ground. (United Nations 2010, paras 20–22)

These findings are revealing. They do not call into question the insight animating the creation of the Commission itself, that peacebuilding requires an integrated and holistic approach, but suggest, rather, that such an approach needs more than logistical attention. Yet even in its recognition that more is needed (United Nations 2010, para. 13), the co-facilitators of the review seem conflicted about the nature of the problem. They recognize that '[t]he existence of a single strategic document does not guarantee that all actors will act in accordance with its priorities' (United Nations 2010, para. 58). However, the problem, as they see it, is not in the singular focus on practical coordination but rather on the failure in support and enforcement of such coordination: '[t]he Commission must use its political weight to seek to align the various actors behind the same overarching

---

1. Alex Boraine (2012), then Chairperson of the International Center for Transitional Justice, addressed a United Nations Panel on 'the essential nature of both peace and justice in post-conflict countries, and the critical issue of sequencing efforts to these ends, while keeping in mind justice as the goal'. See also Roht-Arriaza and Mariezcurrena (2006).

objectives' (United Nations 2010, para. 58). There is also some hint in the review that more than political power may be needed to achieve the goals of the Commission. '[W]e emphasize that the exercise will not succeed unless it is infused with a renewed commitment and a strengthened sense of engagement. Change must be psychological as well as institutional' (United Nations 2010, para. 167). Such psychological change, it would seem, requires more than renewed commitment to practical solutions, it speaks to the need for new ways of understanding peacebuilding and the relationships between the various elements of peace, justice and development.[2] A relational approach revises the conceptual framework in which we understand these elements and their relationship to one another in a way that questions apparent tensions and grounds integrative and holistic strategies.

Restorative Justice: A Relational Theory

Much of the consideration of justice in the literature on post-conflict and peacebuilding takes a narrow view of justice as the demand for a particular approach or manifestation of individual accountability usually through criminal trials and punishment (or sometimes pursued through civil and administrative penalties such as tort/lustration/reparation). This invites debate as to whether justice must be sacrificed, scaled back or compromised to secure other values, notably peace or security. Others take the position that justice should be valued and pursued regardless of the cost or consequences that may follow. On this account the doing of justice has independent moral significance or is viewed as essential to legitimate, meaningful or lasting peace in the long run even if its contribution is not immediate or obvious.

Restorative justice has garnered increased attention over the last decade and a half in post-conflict contexts as an alternative approach or model to deal with issues of accountability and/or reparation; that is, with the operational justice dimension of transitions and peacebuilding. This view is premised on an understanding of restorative justice as either alternative justice *practice* or as an alternative conception of criminal justice. Others have claimed that restorative justice is actually less concerned with justice than with peace and thus ought to be pursued alongside or following 'real' justice understood in terms of retributive justice models. In so far as restorative justice has been pursued in place of other justice mechanisms, restorative justice has been criticized as, at best, partial justice and, at worse, a sacrifice of justice.

All of these understandings and applications of restorative justice fail to appreciate restorative justice as a comprehensive theory of justice and thus miss its full significance and potential for post-conflict contexts and more broadly for

---

2. Daniel Philpott and I sought to offer such a new framework for peacebuilding as part of a recent project shared at the International Symposium on Restorative Justice, Reconciliation and Peace-building in New York (2011) and which will be the subject of an upcoming edited collection.

peacebuilding. Restorative justice, conceived as a relational theory of justice, is able to serve as a conceptual frame for peacebuilding and its interrelated aspects. It is able to move beyond the limited role of justice in relation to peacebuilding. It broadens the concern of justice beyond simply advocating different processes or institutional alternatives to fulfil the task of ensuring individual accountability, a task evident in the familiar focus on the debate between truth commissions and trials. Although a relational approach to peacebuilding will surely have some institutional and operational implications, it is not only or primarily concerned with this work. Rather, a relational theory of justice has implications for thinking about and doing the work of peacebuilding broadly conceived. On this account, justice encompasses not only how to respond to particular wrongful conduct but also to injustice more generally and with the goal of promoting and sustaining just relations.

This refocusing of justice invites a reconsideration of the tensions some see within peacebuilding. Such tensions pit justice as a competitor if not a threat to peace (and vice versa), at least in the immediate aftermath of conflict. Likewise, the relationships between justice and development is cast as a competition for which of these has moral primacy and what resources ought to be invested to achieve these. As discussed in the introduction, such tensions are often resolved by resorting to priority sequencing—holding off development until justice is done or requiring justice before peace can be built. In each case, justice is limited to individual accountability generally achieved through retributive justice. On this account, the relationship among the component elements of peacebuilding is an uneasy one filled with tension and potential conflict. The experience of post-conflict contexts and the UN Peacebuilding Commission calls out for a more integrated and holistic account of peacebuilding, one that can ease tensions and reflect the deep interconnected relationship of peace, justice and development. Restorative justice and the relational framework it offers for the work of peacebuilding challenges the logic of silos and takes sequencing to be an inadequate approach to understanding the component aspects of peacebuilding. It makes clear that security, peace negotiations, justice, development and so on all share a common focus on building the just relationships required for peace that is meaningful and sustainable into the future.

An overview of the relational theory of justice that restorative justice offers is essential to appreciate its potential for framing peacebuilding and the relation-ship of its key elements: peace, justice and development (Llewellyn 2006a, b). Restorative justice is best understood, I suggest, as grounded in feminist relational theory. By virtue of this foundation, restorative justice can be understood as a feminist conception of justice. As such, it is particularly promising for assuring that peacebuilding in all of its component parts of peace, justice and development is attuned to the needs of gender justice. This is not to claim that restorative justice is justice concerned only with the needs of women, but rather that it is able to provide what is essential for gender justice: a theory of justice that takes as its starting point our embodied and relational nature as human beings. Restorative justice is grounded in an understanding of the self as constituted in and through relationships with others. It does not glorify relationships as a 'good' in and of themselves but, rather, claims that relationship is an unavoidable fact about how we live, who we are and how we are formed, informed and reformed. This claim, about the human self, should not be mistaken for social determinism. Our choices and actions are not dictated wholly by the sum of our relationships or relational influences. On a relational account, individuals retain agency. We can still choose for ourselves, but what a relational theory of the self makes clear is that we cannot make or realize our choices by ourselves and our choices have implications for others (Llewellyn 2011). Thus, relational theory does not focus on the collective at the expense of, or in contrast/conflict with, the individual. It offers, instead, a relational picture of the individual, one that places relationship at the core as fundamental and formative.

Recognition that relationality is an unavoidable truth of who we are demands careful and significant attention to relationships and their implications for us. Relationships can be positive or negative and, in so far as we are interested in securing conditions in which individuals can be well and flourish, we need to pay close attention to the character and quality of relationship required. We know from lived experience the sorts of relationships that are antithetical to well-being and flourishing because they cause harm. They are relationships marked by oppression, violence, neglect, abuse and so on. From this experience we have come to know the quality of relationship needed for well-being and flourishing. I have described this as 'equality of relationship' and by this I mean relationships marked by equal respect, concern and dignity (Llewellyn 2011). These values and their importance are not new to us. Indeed, they ground the very tenets of protection for human rights (international and domestic). Enter justice. Under-stood relationally, justice is concerned precisely with the state or nature of our relationships, and injustice and wrong are understood in terms of the harm caused to individuals in relationship with others and in the connections between and among them. Equality of relationship—the equality of respect, concern and dignity that it entails—represents the criterion for just relationships, which is the goal of justice understood relationally. It is this goal to which the restoration of relationships is aimed in restorative justice. On this account, respect, concern and dignity are rooted in our *relational* rather than *rational* nature, as is the case for liberal justice.

The equality at which justice is aimed in this account is relational as well.[3] To claim that justice is, at its core, about relational equality is not to say simply that it is concerned with equality of treatment or outcome for individuals (although this would be desirable). Relational equality is a more fundamental commitment to the nature of relationship between and among parties. Under-standing equality this way makes it easier to see how restorative justice is concerned with equality. It does not reduce matters of justice (and injustice)

---

3. My account is indebted to Christine Koggel's notion of relational equality (1998) in which she distinguishes a relational account from formal and substantive approaches in the liberal tradition.

simply to those of inequality or equality, in the sense in which we understand them in our Western liberal legal tradition. It is not concerned, for example, with the equality that some retributive theories of justice seek through an evening of the score between wrongdoer and victims by inflicting harm against the wrongdoer (typically through isolating punishment) in even measure to that done to the victim.

By contrast, relational justice problematizes the issue of what set of practices can or should be utilized towards the goal of restoring equality in the context of the relationships involved. It demands concrete consideration of the needs and capacities of each party to realize equality of relationship. For a relational theory of justice, then, equality cannot be achieved by ensuring the same treatment or equal measures of benefits or burdens or even identical outcomes for individuals. Instead, equality must be understood and achieved through attention to the nature of the relationships in and through which selves exist. On this under-standing, the interests and concerns of justice align with those of peace and development. Justice is fundamentally concerned with just relationship as the basis for lasting and sustainable peace and with the concrete and contextualized conditions required to realize such relationships.

Restorative Justice and Sen's Idea of Justice

In his recent work *The Idea of Justice*, Amartya Sen (2009) directly considers the implications of a contextual account of justice in relation to development. There are reasons to argue that Sen's is not a relational theory of justice—or at least that Sen does not intend it as such given his focus on the individual as the unit of analysis and his concern with comparing and contrasting individual interests with collective ones.[4] Yet despite the clear influence of liberal individualism, there are aspects of Sen's theory that resonate with, if not reflect, aspects of the relational theory of justice I advocate as a conceptual frame for peacebuilding. Just how relational Sen's idea of justice is awaits another venue.

In his work on the idea of justice, Sen explicitly considers the fundamental relationship between development and justice. The idea of justice he defends shares a core concern of development theory and policy: addressing and alleviating real injustices in the world. Development, on Sen's account, cannot be measured 'merely in terms of enhancement of inanimate objects of convenience, such as a rise in the GNP (or personal incomes), or industrialization' (2009, p. 346). Rather, development is, for Sen, more broadly concerned with human lives—that is with what people are free to do or are capable of doing on the basis of such development. However, this broader view of development does not render enhancement of GNP, industrialization or other 'enhancements of inanimate objects of convenience' irrelevant to development. Indeed, develop-ment must be, Sen advises, concerned with economic poverty because it can

---

4. This issue has received some attention in the literature (Koggel 2003; Hill 2003; Gore 1997).

have a real effect on people's lives and freedoms (p. 346). Sen is, thus, focused, as is a restorative approach, on the outcome of justice processes. Restorative justice measures justice (and justice processes) by their contribution to the realization of relationships of equality between and among the individuals and communities involved. For Sen, justice is concerned with the reduction of injustice in the lived experience of those concerned. As such, attention must be paid to the contextualized, embodied and embedded human experience of justice and injustices. Sen contrasts this focus on injustices in the real world with the traditional concern in contemporary justice theory with 'perfect justice' as reflected and achieved by just institutions or social arrangements (p. 86). The weakness of such an approach, Sen argues, is the lack of attention it pays to the outcomes and implications of those institutional arrangements for the lived reality of people. Restorative justice similarly focuses attention on the contexts of injustice but, unlike Sen, it uses the lens of the *relationships* in and through which we live as the way to assess injustices.

Neither Sen's idea of justice nor a relational one take as a measure of justice its achievement or success as compared with some ideal. Rather, Sen makes it clear that justice seeks and can only achieve something *better* (in terms of less injustice or more justice) but not perfection in an ideal sense (p. 100). Relational theory also explains the need to think of justice in concrete terms, as it exists in the world. Justice consists, then, in addressing injustices in their concrete and contextual manifestations, not through comparison with pre-determined social arrangements/institutions. It is worth noting that this feature of restorative justice frustrates many who seek instruction as to what exactly just social relationships look like—looking for that picture of perfect justice that Sen also rejects. In fact, relational theory invites us to think about justice in ways that our current justice language makes difficult. We speak commonly of seeing justice 'done' or 'served up' or 'achieved'. Relational theory requires an adjustment in the very way that we understand the work that justice requires. The question of what justice requires, then, cannot be met by standard and formulaic answers but, rather, must take into account what is needed in a particular context to achieve just relationships between and among the parties involved. This is work that, like the relationships it seeks to achieve, is dynamic and fluid. Thus, it may be more appropriate to adjust our discourse from talking about justice 'done' to 'doing justice'. This is not to suggest that relational justice is purely procedural in nature. In its idea of equality of relationship, relational justice offers a substantive goal or end state. The shift in language, however, acknowledges that relational justice does not identify justice with any one set of practices (or perfect institutional arrangements) but, rather, requires the input and participation of those involved to understand the nature of the harm to relationships in order to determine how to respond.

While rejecting a focus on perfect institutional arrangements, on a restorative approach to justice, as on Sen's account, it is still important to consider institutions. However, 'we have to see institutions that *promote* justice, rather than treating the institutions as themselves manifestations of justice, which would reflect a kind of institutionally fundamentalist view' (Sen 2009, p. 82; emphasis in original). Institutional arrangements, then, are not the objective of justice but rather are mechanisms in and through which just relationships might be enabled and supported (or undermined as the case may be). As Sen notes, those who see justice in terms of perfect institutional arrangements tend to presume human behaviour will conform to such institutional norms. For Sen, and for restorative justice, people need to come to know what is required to realize justice in the world. This requires a more complex approach that pays attention to the need for processes and institutions that are contextual and flexible to account for and accommodate differing human needs and behaviours and facilitate justice work. Restorative justice reflects this complexity in its attention to process and institutions not as the end of justice but as essential for the encounter, dialogue and deliberation that justice requires. Through such processes restorative justice is able to take account of the significance and complexity of the interconnected webs of relationships in and through which we exist and come to define and understand both ourselves and what justice requires. A relational theory of justice requires processes that are inclusive and participatory—especially of those individuals affected by or with a concern for the outcome of a matter. Through dialogical processes, parties are able to understand harms resulting from a wrong and/or recognize broader injustices, and arrive at a plan for addressing the harms/injustices with a view to realizing equality of relationship in the future. Through broad inclusion, such processes are able to ensure the appropriate balance between macro- and micro-justice issues and avoid sacrificing the needs and interests of one for the other.

On Sen's account, democracy is about more than voting; it entails 'government by discussion' (2009, p. 324). Sen looks to public reasoning as a way to determine the requirements of justice in specific contexts. Restorative justice processes are similarly committed to ensuring space for public reasoning. They are democratic in the sense that they strive to ensure that those affected can participate in the processes of decision making about how to do justice in a particular situation. It is, thus, not sufficient for parties simply to be included, they must be given the opportunity to *participate* in a meaningful way, which includes, but is not limited to, taking part in a dialogue about the requirements of justice. While Sen acknowledges the important relationship between justice and democracy, I would argue that a focus on just relationship can better illustrate the importance of participation and dialogue in the very understanding of what justice requires in specific contexts of unjust relationship.

Sen's defence of non-ideal theory, theory that emerges from public reasoning and dialogue within a specific context, with the goal of measuring injustices and determining how to alleviate them, has made Sen susceptible to the objection that he needs to specify and list particular capabilities by which we could measure the presence, absence or amount of justice. A version of this objection against restorative justice is the call for precision in the form of relationships that will count as restored (read: just). 'Tell us', such critics call, 'what is the model of restored relationship—what does it look like?' Restorative justice can only respond 'It depends' and offer a process to take into account that upon which it depends. But this is not a regrettable answer for restorative justice, or for Sen's account, for justice on these accounts is not abstract. It is concerned about justice as it is lacking or realized in the world. Democratic processes do not, in and of themselves, satisfy justice but, rather, are essential to ascertaining what justice requires in concrete terms. Justice does not depend on democracy but rather on the understanding that is made possible through democratic deliberations (Llewellyn 2006a).

Sen's consideration of the relationship between democracy and development is also helpful in illuminating a perceived tension between them that mirrors a tension often posited for restorative justice between justice and peace. Addressing such tensions is key if restorative justice is to succeed in its claim for a more integrated and holistic approach to peacebuilding. Sen explains the concern in this way: 'The observation of a handful of such examples led rapidly to something of a general theory: democracies do quite badly in facilitating development, compared with what authoritarian regimes can achieve' (2009, p. 345). Responding to this concern requires, Sen argues, attention to the content of the ideas of both democracy and development at work. In so far as the argument against the positive relationship between democracy and development relies upon the notion that elections do not ensure economic growth, Sen suggests that the objection misunderstands his claim. Rather, a broader understanding of both democracy and development makes a different case for their relationship. It goes beyond their external links to a constitutive connection (p. 346). It is also important to note that Sen claims that the case in favour of the relatively detrimental effect of democracy on development (and thereby the relationship of justice to development) is overstated and unsupported by the evidence. A fuller cross-country comparison than that offered by his critics does not bear out the claim that democracy slows economic growth (p. 348). Restorative justice parallels this argument by claiming that justice does not and need not slow peacebuilding.

Restorative Justice and the False Dichotomy of Peace versus Justice

I have been suggesting that a restorative approach to peacebuilding stands to address one of the most significant perceived dilemmas in peacebuilding: the choice of peace versus justice. Restorative justice is sometimes invoked to ease this tension between justice and peace. Understanding restorative justice through the framework of transitional justice, however, limits the full potential and capacity of restorative justice to offer a way out of the justice versus peace dichotomy. Generally, restorative justice is presented by transitional justice scholars as either the measure or part of justice that is available given the complex set of circumstances that often exist in transitional contexts. On this view, restorative justice represents justice to the extent possible given the circumstances. Sometimes it is characterized as justice for victims and, at other times, it is the justice available when the 'full' justice of prosecution and punishment cannot be undertaken.[5] Other advocates of transitional justice suggest that restorative justice is a kind or type of justice that is most appropriate for transitional periods. On this account (which is less common) restorative justice is viewed as full justice for transitions. However, implicit in this view (and sometime explicit) is the claim that this is a compromise of justice nonetheless brought about by the particular set of circumstances faced in transitional contexts. Restorative justice is thus justice for transitions but has no implications, on this account, for the meaning of justice beyond (Llewellyn 2006a).

The best response to the challenge that the justice versus peace dilemma poses to the integrated and holistic approach to peacebuilding that restorative justice offers asks us to attend to the constitutive relationship between justice and peace (a move similar to the constitutive relationship that Sen draws between democracy and development). Understood more broadly, as a relational theory of justice, restorative justice is neither partial justice nor is it a special *kind* of justice for extraordinary circumstances. Rather, transitional contexts may be significant for this idea of justice by virtue of the clarity they offer about the nature of justice sometimes obscured in more normal times: that the restoration of relationships is at the heart of justice (Llewellyn 2006b). Restorative justice is thus capable of offering a way out of the dilemma between peace and justice. On a relational account, justice is fundamentally concerned with and oriented towards the establishment of equality of relationship which is constitutive of lasting and sustainable peace.

Moreover, broadening the understanding of justice does not suggest that individual accountability is irrelevant to peace. Indeed, just as levels of income are relevant to an assessment of development so too is individual accountability relevant to peace. No regard for individual accountability for harm would obviously put peace at risk since it would enable continued and future harm to individuals and their relationships. But restorative justice does not require a choice between individual accountability and the broader vision of justice as concerned with restored relationships. On a restorative account the two are not separable. Where an individual has committed a wrong the harm caused is addressed in terms of the related harm to relationships. Critics are right to assert that the restoration of relationships, at which justice aims, and which is, in turn, the bedrock of peace, cannot be brought through impunity (Llewellyn 2001). However, critics are wrong to see this as a weakness of restorative justice. The evidence shows that restorative justice does not sacrifice individual account-ability for peace.

---

5. Reference to the retributive justice of prosecution and punishment as 'normal', 'full', 'ordinary' or 'proper' justice is common within the literature on transitional justice. See, for example, Goldstone (2000, p. ix); Shriver (2001, p. 1); and Allen (1999, p. 315).

In fact, restorative justice may be better suited for meaningful accountability for a few reasons. First, restorative processes engage offenders in a process that enables and encourages them to accept responsibility and to play an active role in addressing the harm related to their actions. Contrary to the critics' claim that restorative justice is tantamount to impunity or soft justice, it seems actually to demand more of wrongdoers than the passive acceptance of punishment (or, as is more often the case, the active denial of responsibility) prompted by adversarial criminal justice processes. Restorative justice is, thus, able to do better than *holding* offenders to account by facilitating the assumption of responsibility by offenders themselves that is essential for participation in future peaceful social relations. Second, individual accountability can be better understood within a restorative process committed to understanding fully the contexts and causes of a wrong. This more complex and nuanced understanding of responsibility is essential to building sustainable and lasting peace in the future. Third, the evidence rests in favour of restorative justice in terms of compliance and deterrence.[6] Restorative justice, then, is not only constitutive of peace but also better able than narrower conceptions of justice to secure peace.

Dispelling the perceived tensions between democracy and development and justice and peace illuminates the difference a new lens on justice brings to our settled assumptions about the tensions inherent in the work of peacebuilding. It demonstrates the possibility and promise of framing peacebuilding in a way that understands the relationships between its component parts of peace, justice and development.

Conclusion

Restorative justice is capable of offering the conceptual framework that peacebuilding needs in order to move beyond operational strategies to manage the tensions and relationships between peace, justice and development. Feminist relational theory grounds a conception of justice that moves beyond the narrow focus on justice as merely an element or stage of peacebuilding to an understanding of peacebuilding as the work of building sustainable just social relationships. Justice on this account requires accountability and responsibility not as the end of justice but as elements of the broader task of addressing injustice and establishing better relationships that reflect the values of equality of relationship. This relational lens can be applied to all the elements of peacebuilding to offer a better understanding and reorientation of their respective and collective interrelationship. For the work of justice, as it has

---

6. Note that the evidence is largely in the context of domestic criminal justice. See, for example, Sherman and Strang (2007). However, experience in post-conflict societies has shown the weakness of criminal justice in that restorative responses have often also been practically better able to ensure accountability in the wake of the inaction or inability of criminal justice to deal with the volume of cases.

been narrowly pursued, the reorientation entails a move away from processes that focus solely on individual culpability and rely on adversarial processes to produce truth and remedy. It might mean a move away from the traditional Western justice model of prosecution and punishment towards restorative institutions that facilitate inclusive and participatory processes aimed at meaningful accountability through expression of responsibility and participation in making reparation for harm. A similar shift would be entailed for development from the traditional (possibly still mainstream) view of development aimed at economic attainment through industrialization (and often Westernization) towards a focus on the processes that can enhance the freedoms sought by development as Sen envisions it.

Peacebuilding, with its elements of peace, justice and development, cannot be satisfied by crafting perfectly just social institutions (or UN architectures). To be sure, institutions and processes will be important, but only in so far as they can facilitate the relationships needed in particular contexts to enable and promote human flourishing and contribute to lasting and sustainable peace.

Acknowledgements

I am grateful for the helpful comments I received from participants at the IDEA conference at Bryn Mawr. I am particularly indebted to Christine Koggel for her support and encouragement. Thanks are also owed to Dan Van Ness, John Braithwaite and Dan Philpott for the insights and inspiration they have offered.

References

Allen, J. (1999) 'Balancing Justice and Social Unity: Political Theory and the Idea of a Truth and Reconciliation Commission', *University of Toronto Law Journal*, Vol. 49, no. 3, pp. 315–53.

Annan, K. (2005) *In Larger Freedom: Towards Development, Security and Human Rights for All*, United Nations, New York, available at: <http://www.un.org/largerfreedom/chap3.htm> (accessed 5 October 2006).

Boraine, A. (2012) 'Experts Discuss the UN Approach to Transitional Justice', United Nations Rule of Law, available at: <www.unrol.org/article.aspx?article_id=70> (accessed 26 March 2012).

Goldstone, R. (2000) 'Foreword', in *Looking Back, Reaching Forward: Reflections on the Truth and Reconciliation Commission of South Africa*, eds C. Villa-Vicencio & W. Verwoerd, University of Cape Town Press, Cape Town, pp. viii–xiii.

Gore, C. (1997) 'Irreducibly Social Goods and the Informational Basis of Amartya Sen's Capability Approach', *Journal of International Development*, Vol. 9, no. 2, pp. 235–50.

Hill, M. T. (2003) 'Development as Freedom', *Feminist Economics*, Vol. 9, no. 2–3, pp. 117–35.

International Symposium on Restorative Justice, Reconciliation and Peacebuilding (2011) New York University School of Law, available at: <www.iilj.org/rjrp/video.asp> (accessed 27 June 2012).

Koggel, C. (1998) *Perspectives on Equality: Constructing a Relational Theory*, Rowman & Littlefield, Lanham, MD.

Koggel, C. (2003) 'Globalization and Women's Paid Work: Expanding Freedom?', *Feminist Economics*, Vol. 9, nos 2–3, pp. 163–83.

Llewellyn, J. (2001) 'Just Amnesty and Private International Law', in *Torture as Tort: Comparative Perspectives on the Development of Transnational Human Rights Litigation*, ed. C. Scott, Hart, Oxford, pp. 567–600.

Llewellyn, J. (2006a) 'Restorative Justice in Transitions and Beyond: The Justice Potential of Truth Telling Mechanisms for Post-peace Accord Societies', in *Telling the Truths: Truth Telling and Peace Building in Post-conflict Societies*, ed. T. Borer, Notre Dame Press, Notre Dame, pp. 83–114.

Llewellyn, J. (2006b) 'Truth Commissions and Restorative Justice', in *Handbook of Restorative Justice*, eds G. Johnstone & D. Van Ness, Willan, Cullompton, pp. 351–71.

Llewellyn, J. (2011) 'Restorative Justice: Thinking Relationally about Justice', in *Being Relational: Reflections on Relational Theory and Health Law*, eds J. Downie & J. Llewellyn, UBC Press, Vancouver, pp. 89–108.

Roht-Arriaza, N. & Mariezcurrena, J. (eds) (2006) *Transitional Justice in the Twenty-first Century: Beyond Truth versus Justice*, Cambridge University Press, Cambridge and New York.

Sen, A. (2009) *The Idea of Justice*, Harvard University Press, Cambridge, MA.

Sherman, L. & Strang, H. (2007) *Restorative Justice: The Evidence*, Smith Institute, London.

Shriver, Jr., D. W. (2001) 'Truth Commissions and Judicial Trials: Complementary or Antagonistic Servants of Public Justice?', *Journal of Law and Religion*, Vol. 16, no. 1, pp. 1–33.

United Nations (2010) *Review of the United Nations Peacebuilding Architecture*, United Nations A/64/868–S/2010/393 (July).

Partiality Based on Relational Responsibilities: Another Approach to Global Ethics

Joan C. Tronto

Universalistic claims about the nature of justice are presumed to require larger commitments from a global perspective than partialist claims. This essay departs from standard partialist accounts by anchoring partialist claims in a different account of the nature of responsibility. In contrast to substantive responsibility, which is akin to an obligation and derived from principles, relational responsibilities grow out of relationships and their complex intertwining. While such accounts of responsibility are less clear cut, they will prove in the long run to be more valuable in thinking about global ethics. I illustrate this point by considering the moral issue surrounding abandoned relationships. The approach offered here—partiality that rests upon relational responsibilities—makes the responsibilities owed by those in higher income countries towards lower income countries much richer and more complex than is usually presumed.

Introduction

Usual discussions of global justice strive to apply liberal or cosmopolitan notions that invoke our common humanity to provoke those in higher income countries to contribute to people in lower income countries. There is an admirable body of literature that attempts to appeal to people's better selves and to share their wealth with those less fortunate around the globe. For example, in *One World*, Peter Singer proposes that

> as a public policy likely to produce good consequences...anyone who has enough money to spend on the luxuries and frivolities so common in affluent societies should give at least 1 cent in every dollar of their income to those who have

trouble getting enough to eat, clean water to drink, shelter from the elements, and basic health care. (Singer 2002, p. 194)

Thomas Pogge (2008) has argued that from a justice perspective, wealthy countries should be forced to accept responsibility for the injustices of global poverty that they helped to create and continue to perpetuate in their global economic and political activities. For Pogge, rich states' greater control over the institutions of the global political economy stand as an indictment in their ongoing and continuing creation of global poverty. Feminist thinkers such as Carol Gould (2004) and Alison Jaggar (2005) have also argued that current arrangements that insulate people in the Global North from the harm that their actions inflict upon others are unjust. Yet despite the force of these arguments, somehow they have failed to move citizens, publics, politicians, and states to do enough.

Most writers who advance partialist accounts of responsibility do so with the hope of limiting broad claims for global responsibility. My claim here is quite different. This paper eschews the claim that we owe support to others simply because, like us, they are human and their suffering, or their experience of depending upon care, should therefore matter. Thinking from such a perspective, the arguments are both too demanding and insufficiently demanding. They are too demanding because, if we take them seriously, they raise a problem of limits: what is the proper response to others' suffering? If people are really suffering, then why should Singer's modest 1 percent contribution suffice? Perhaps those in higher income countries should abandon entirely their profligate lifestyle. Caught by not knowing what is 'enough', too many people solve the moral issues by resorting to doing nothing. Instead, I shall argue that stronger, and more action-inducing, partialist claims can be made if we think in terms of relational responsibilities towards others around the globe. In order to make this claim, I need first to explain the nature of relational responsibility, and then to suggest how it can produce such strong claims. On the basis of the nature of relational responsibilities themselves, I argue that the moral harm from abandoned relationships is the serious ground upon which deep and profound obligations to others around the globe are now owed. In the end, responsibility understood relationally provides a stronger basis for and gives more content and meaning to claims about what various people around the globe owe to each other.

Relational Responsibility

Most contemporary accounts of responsibility treat the term 'responsibility' as if it were synonymous with terms such as 'duty' or 'obligation'. For example, Samuel Scheffler's *Boundaries and Allegiances* (2001) equates 'distinctive responsibilities' with 'special obligations' (p. 36) and later with 'associative duties' (pp. 48–65). The standard discussion of responsibility revolves around the substance of what the actor (whether an individual or collective actor, such as a corporation or state) intends and around the effects of the action. By this account, responsibilities in relationships derive their force from a set of claims made about the formal *properties* of relationships. Given their emphasis on such properties, I shall call this the 'substantive' account of responsibility; it matches the kind of rational deduction about 'duties' that derive from substantive principles of justice.[1] For example, a claim that family members are responsible for meeting the caring needs of children in their household rests upon the formal claim that the property of having children makes one responsible for them.

This paper, instead, draws upon a notion of relational responsibility. Feminist thinkers, among others, have thought about how understanding the world *relationally* transforms such concepts as autonomy (McKenzie & Stoljar 2000) and equality (Koggel 1998). Drawing inspiration from the writings of Soran Reader (2003), I describe an account of *relational responsibility*.[2]

The term responsibility, which only entered the English language in the mid-seventeenth century, connotes a kind of 'response', which is, on its face, relational. Reader argues that relations are a particular kind of interaction (and not only among humans but also with other living and inanimate things in the world). By her account, what make relations distinctive are the kinds of engagement of the moral actor with the 'relata'. So, while a person might be a member of the group 'recipients of heart transplants', that status, condition, substantive property does not become a relation until one heart transplant recipient seeks out another, becomes engaged with others similarly situated about how their lives have been affected by their common experience, their initial conversations blossom into a friendship, and so forth (Reader 2003, p. 374). Such relations, and not merely sharing properties, argues Reader, make agents responsible: 'The mark of obligation-constituting features of real relationships is that they are not merely properties that the relata happen to share. Rather, they are properties that literally connect, constituting the relationship. Such features both connect and obligate agents' (p. 370). Thus, Reader's agents have voluntaristic qualities to some extent that make them responsible, but not all responsibilities arise voluntarily. This is so since they may have been the relata, that is, the object of a relation created by someone else; for example, an infant does not choose her caregivers but is, nonetheless, deeply related to them.

---

1. To fill in aspects of this substantive account, see, for example, Leib's view of the 'four central grounds' of responsibility: what an agent causes, what she chooses, what she identifies with, and what sort of character she has (2006). Reader's account might fall into category three, but not all of Reader's identifications are voluntary (2003).

2. It would require a separate paper to catalog the various useful ways in which responsibility has been subdivided and to explain how this account of relational responsibility differs from all of them. Among works that have been especially useful to me in thinking about this question are Feinberg (1980); Haskell (1998); Scheffler (1997, 2001); Smiley (1992); Walker (2007); Young (2006).

Reader specifies that relations that lead to responsibility can arise in a number of ways. They can arise from presence, biology, history, practice, environment, shared projects, institutions, play, trade, conversation, and other 'less structured interactions'. The resulting responsibilities will vary, but they vary not because there is a substantive moral principle that describes their value. Rather, they vary with the depth of the relationship that exists: 'obligations are also stronger if the relationship is fuller' (p. 377).

Reader's account of relations thus recognizes that responsibilities are necessarily partial, yet, depending upon the agents' deeds and activities, they can be quite far-reaching and myriad. In this regard, she claims, partialists are correct to see that relationships matter, but wrong 'in the kinds of relational properties they have hitherto singled out' (p. 370). She distinguishes her account from other limiting, partialists accounts by noting how broadly she sees partialist obligations in daily life, by 'seeing moral obligation as a part of not just some but all relationships, and in accounting for the way moral obligations diminish, and thereby accommodating the impartialist intuition that strangers may obligate us morally' (p. 379). But strangers do not obligate us simply by sharing with us the substantive property of being human. Some form of relation—either presence, biological, historical, or institutional ties, or some other form of 'interaction'—exists in order to create a relation and, thus, a responsibility.[3]

Other scholars have also devised relational models of responsibility. Iris Young's 'social connection model' of responsibility (2006) argued that all agents who contribute by their actions to the structural processes that produce injustice have responsibilities to work to remedy these injustices. She distinguished the social connection model from a 'liability' model, and allowed that in legal proceedings the liability model still has an important role to play. Writing about the example of college students boycotting the production of licensed college wear in sweatshops led Young to realize that the 'liability' model was inadequate. One can say that the sweatshop owner had committed a moral wrong, but the response 'at least they have some work' is also somewhat persuasive. Young recognized, as had Marion Smiley (1992) before her, that trying to parse out who is wrong and deserves blame does not solve the problem of irresponsible action. Drawing upon her career-long meditations on the complicated relationships of agency and social structure, Young recognized the more complex nature of 'structural injustice', in which, though we can see an ongoing and continuing social injustice, the actions of particular others may not be traced through complex social institutions to clear causal paths. As a result, Young argued, everyone involved bears some, albeit different, level of responsibility. She averred that different conditions of power, privilege, interest, and capacities for collective action might make some more responsible and others less responsible. Thus, while everyone who perceives a situation of structural

---

3. In one of Reader's examples a stranger falls down in front of another person on the street. In this case, presence creates a relationship. Now, whether presence does create a relationship here is actually a *political question*. Consider places where the 'street' is an expected site of danger and the reaction might be different.

injustice has a responsibility to address it, 'By virtue of this structural positioning, different agents have different opportunities and capacities, can draw on different kinds and amounts of resources, or face different levels of constraint with respect to processes that can contribute to structural change' (Young 2006, p. 126). Young then added the obvious point that such complexities cross national borders to explain how responsibilities might also cross national borders.[4]

The most far-reaching account of relational responsibility is that offered by Margaret Urban Walker (2007). Walker's concept of responsibility grows out of a meta-ethical critique: moral understandings, she observes, are 'mainly about moral epistemology, that is, about the nature, source, and justification of moral knowledge' (p. 4). Walker distinguishes two kinds of meta-ethics: the theoretical-juridical model and the expressive-collaborative model. The former is concerned with elucidating clear moral principles following standard rules of philosophical practice and the latter denies that any moral actor's position, including the philosopher's, is superior to others. Instead, only through moral practices—the expression, agreement, and collaboration about the meaning of morality in any community—does moral life take form. Walker calls the practice of the expressive-collaborative meta-ethic an 'ethics of responsibility': 'An "ethics of responsibility" as a normative view would try to put people and responsibilities in the right places with respect to each other' (p. 84). As a result, morality becomes 'a social negotiation in real time, where members of a community of roughly or largely shared moral beliefs try to refine understanding, extend consensus, and eliminate conflict among themselves' (p. 71).

As an account of global responsibility, Walker's is still aspirational, in part because we may not see ourselves as a global or cross-national moral community and in part because there are still very few institutions for placing us in relation to others so that we may resolve our global responsibilities. (It may not be surprising that such institutions are emerging first around legal questions such as criminal blame and human rights.) Walker remained, in *Moral Understandings*, open to the possibility that traditional moral theory can provide us with useful insights. In *Moral Repair* (2006), Walker often uses more traditional accounts of liability-assignment as a way to think about our current moral situation. Nevertheless, given its emphasis on the relationships that exist among moral

---

4. At first glance, Young's model may seem to be different from Reader's account that assumes the agent will recognize the connection with the relata and, indeed, that the connection constitutes both the relationship and the obligation. This seems far removed from an engagement with notions of 'structural injustice'. But perhaps a better way to read Young's account is to see the 'social connection' as a challenge about what 'matters'—what connects us—in our lives. The sweatshop example allows Young to expand the notion of fashion and the kinds of connections and meanings it creates. For fashionistas, having a sophisticated sense of style may be a central part of one's identity. Even people who do not care about fashion are still concerned with it; to show up inappropriately clothed for class, work, or social engagements disrupts social interactions. A person poorly attired might be ashamed, embarrassed, or disregarded. Even if we may not want to acknowledge this connection, we are tied to the person who makes our clothing. Unlike the somewhat clearer accounts of our responsibilities that flow from a more fixed account of justice, these accounts of relational responsibility provide greater room for digging down into the concrete details of interrelationship.

parties, Walker's account of responsibility also fits within this second, relational not substantive, account of responsibility.[5]

Advantages of Using a Relational Approach to Responsibility

Having distinguished these two forms of responsibility, we can now see how they differently inform partial moral judgments. In order to make moral judgments from the standpoint of substantive responsibility, associative duties require that one return to the principles of justice and the types of substantive claims that can be made. Like Walker's theoretico-juridical meta-ethics, partialist theories of substantive responsibility posit certain substantive responsibilities as central and deduce proper moral action from them. This more juridical account of responsibility differs fundamentally from relational responsibility, where the fact of being alive and the nature of human vulnerability places one in relationships and thus already in the midst of relationships that produce responsibilities. A relational account of responsibility thus requires a different set of facts and circumstances to make moral judgments that involve the details of real ongoing relationships. It thus goes beyond the perspective of choice or other attributes of individuals in assigning responsibility. This difference is significant when people consider their place in the world and their connections, and responsibilities, to others. It reverses a frequently made assumption—as Fabrizio Turoldo and Michael Barilan put it, 'Caring for anything is the first bud of responsibility; if cultivated, it may grow and develop' (2008, p. 120). Rather, we might say that responsibilities *already exist* whenever caring needs have been met.

Once we begin to notice that assigning, accepting, deferring, deflecting, and meeting responsibility involves power, some of the important asymmetries of responsibility are revealed. The advantage of the relational approach to responsibility becomes clear once we begin to think about assessing the seriousness of irresponsibility. A standard account of responsibility can make strong claims upon agents to fulfill their responsibilities-as-obligations, which require us to investigate what the agent intended and did. But from a relational approach, it is not simply the agent's voluntarism, or the strength of the causal chain, but the consequence of acting irresponsibly that determines the degree of harm that comes from irresponsibility. Some elements become more important in assessing the harm of irresponsibility. For example, the imbalances of power in relationships between a welfare worker and a client seeking welfare are a serious moral dimension of a responsibility relationship. So too the relative strength of competing responsibilities for caregivers would factor into a judgment when a caregiver ignores or downplays a particular responsibility.

---

5. A related argument is Fiona Robinson's (1999) globalizing care ethics. She directly criticizes the idea that our relationships and responsibilities are contained within the sovereign nation-state. She argues that the nation-state and its containment of obligations of citizenship do not exhaust our morally relevant relationships.

Simply because responsibilities are not universal does not diminish their moral importance. Partial responsibilities are surely more binding upon us than universal obligations. Consider this example: everyone is not responsible for everyone else's care. But in any society, decisions about who cares for whom, how, and why, underpin the way the society or social system is organized. It is an empirical question whether gaps in care exist, and if they do, then a strong case can be made for political action to address them. But one does not need to make a claim about each owing the same to all in order to move such an agenda forward.

One of the problems with substantive partialist theories (such as Scheffler's) is that they have no basis for making assessments about the quality of the relationship that produces the obligation. By such accounts, if one owed an obligation, for example, because of a family relationship, then the quality of the relationship could not affect the degree of responsibility it imposed on one. As Marilyn Friedman observes (1991), one cannot simply say that because a relationship exists it should have special moral status; after all there can be bad relationships and morally indefensible ones. Reader began to provide an answer to this question by pointing out that the constitutive nature of relation-ships also specifies their content and meaning for participants (2003, p. 376). This is likely to be protection against justification for self-serving or bad relationships.

A main objection to basing global ethics on partiality is that it makes it impossible for duties to expand across boundaries. That notion assumes, substantively, that boundaries define the most important forms of relationships. Scheffler (2001) explores such 'associative duties' or 'special responsibilities' as a part of our 'common sense morality' and concludes that the nation-state seems to have a strong hold on the claim for being the legitimate container for such responsibilities. He does so by showing that none of the objections we can raise to such associative obligations, which he characterizes as the voluntarist and the distributive objections to them, completely succeed. Thus, we are left with people's common sense limit to their moral actions; that they abide by the laws in their own society. Hence, partiality ends at a nation's borders.[6]

Scheffler begins from a 'liberal' understanding of responsibilities; his argu-ment presumes that the individual is the appropriate unit from which to engage the question of the nature of responsibility. Scheffler examines some of the tensions between more specific and more general responsibilities. In the end, though, he recognizes that our special responsibilities will appear more 'natural' and thus more concrete to us (2001, chap. 2). Scheffler decries such unjustified partiality, but his analysis provides scant account for how we might address them.

A relational account of responsibility is preferable because it places these conflicts about the nature of responsibility at the heart of the political, social, and epistemological bearings of each and every individual and institution.

---

6. For a different argument about the problem of holding nations accountable over time, see Miller (2004).

Because people and institutions exist within a complex, often competing, set of relations, responsibilities are also likely to be complex and competing. Acting irresponsibly towards one relationship might also grow out of setting higher priorities on other responsibilities. In truth, from this perspective, we will probably seem to be more likely not to meet our responsibilities than to meet them. Thus, the idea of being irresponsible towards some of the responsibilities in our lives will be a matter of course for most humans, not a result of a rare fault. Once we agree that responsibilities have different degrees of depth and different levels of social pull upon us, each person or group can begin to make a more nuanced account of what any responsibility requires and the seriousness of its concomitant irresponsibility.

Finally, relational irresponsibility allows us to bring the question of power imbalances back into the heart of relations of responsibility. In a way, Scheffler has approached the question of unequal power and resources in his 'distributive objection' to special responsibilities. From the outside, he observes that someone left out of a set of special associations may suffer. He also considers the effect of such relationships among the members of an 'In Group'. But his account does not make allowances for a very deep account of such unequal relations, which are, ultimately, probably a majority of the relations in which people find themselves. Nevertheless, relational responsibility recommends itself in that it centers the fact that a relationship may have a profoundly different effect for different parties within a relationship. Two friends may place different weight on the value of their friendship to themselves, an example that may be familiar but not so profound. 'When the United States sneezes, Latin America catches the flu', as the old saw goes, also captures this idea; failure to meet a responsibility within a relationship may affect the parties differently.

Power and Relational Responsibilities in a Global Context

If we wish to think about responsibility in a global context, what is the most promising way for us to understand responsibility? As many philosophers have noted, the strongest alternative that keeps people from taking their global moral responsibilities seriously is the claim that their moral responsibilities end at the boundaries of their own nation-state (see, for example, Singer 2002, p. 195). Partiality is usually understood in this way, and the partial commitments to the nation-state are seen as the strongest of 'special responsibilities'. But there is no reason why an obvious and strong critique of one partial commitment—that to national community—should negate the possible value of all forms of partialist accounts of responsibility. In a way, the claims about relational responsibility developed and defended here are 'partialist'. But though they are not universal, they are far-reaching. If individuals in the Global North do participate in states and other institutions (like corporations), and those institutions cause harm elsewhere, then the individuals are, at least at some level, responsible. The question of how to get citizens to understand that responsibility is still at stake.

One aspect of Scheffler's argument stands out as a response to claims such as those made by Young in defending a 'social connection' model of responsibility. Scheffler observes that the individual citizens, who he sees as overwhelmed by the institutions in which they find themselves, did not choose to be there:

> [T]he global perspective highlights the importance of various large-scale causal processes, and patterns of activity that the individual agent cannot in general control, but within which individual behaviour is nevertheless subsumed in ways that the individual is, at any given time, unlikely to be in a position fully to appreciate. (Scheffler 2001, p. 44)

After he allows that complex actions have unintended consequences and that individuals may not be able to perceive such consequences as the effects of their choices, Scheffler continues:

> By structuring individual choices in the way that they do, these arrangements serve, in effect, to harness and channel human actions: to recruit them as contributors to larger processes that typically have little to do with people's reasons for performing these actions, but which often have profound and far-reaching effects. Frequently, moreover, the individual agents involved, far from intending to participate in the production of these effects, are scarcely even aware that they have done so. (p. 44)

Note that while Scheffler defends an account of agentic-centered responsibility that rests upon a distributive claim, this part of his argument does not. In making this 'voluntarist' critique, Scheffler's conception of responsibility has returned to the other half of the substantive one, to the view of responsibility best characterized by Young as the 'liability model' of responsibility. But surely Scheffler's point is correct; how can we hold people responsible for something that they did not do and cannot even imagine as a consequence of their actions? Even if one benefited from structural injustice, for example, one can argue that one did not ask for, or even know about, the benefits. Here the limits of a substantive, agentic-centered account of responsibility become clear.[7] How can people be held responsible for consequences that they do not understand as connected to them in any way? At the very least, people in the Global North who 'don't know' the effects their governments and global corporations (whose stock they might buy or own through a pension fund) have on the world's poor can be persuaded to see their lack of knowledge as *ignorance*. Ignorance has many meanings, but consider its role in asymmetric relationships. When the more powerful get advantages by ignoring the effect of the relationship on the less powerful, their ignorance proves beneficial.

---

7. Stephen Esquith describes responsibility that arises from the benefits of others' past action as 'bystander responsibility' (2010).

A partialist account of obligations that is based on responsibility but is not relational may extend further than some theorists of partiality want to allow. But they do not extend as far as responsible relational accounts. Consider, for example, the critique of Scheffler and other partialists offered by Ypi *et al.* (2009). They start from the premise that Scheffler offers; namely, that partialist obligations have associative duties. They then argue that, since actions such as colonialism or imposing a dictator on another people, is harm, then one bears a responsibility when one has harmed others. Since associative duties require distributive justice within one's own country, they continue, there is no basis to end these associative duties at one's national border. By this account, then, partialist responsibilities extend quite far and quite broadly. Indeed, they push this argument to its logical limits and assert that since the harms of colonialism extend throughout a colonial network, former colonies (such as the United States) might owe other former colonies (such as Jamaica) through the transitive nature of associative duties (Ypi *et al.* 2009, p. 134). Ending with the stipulation that 'one person's QED is another's reductio' (p. 134), they believe that they have shown that those who would argue for partialist accounts of responsibility actually are caught in a wider set of associative duties than they would want to admit.

While Ypi *et al.* are trying to broaden the global duties that partialists must accept, their argument rests upon their assumptions about associative duties. For Scheffler, there is a somewhat easy answer to their argument. In *Boundaries and Allegiances*, Scheffler denies that associative duties *within* the nation require distributive solutions. Thus, Ypi *et al.*'s argument that, in order to be consistent, Scheffler will have to recognize broader international duties fails. Since they impose their own view of domestic distributive responsibilities on to these partialist accounts, they extend their argument further than it can be stretched.

But from the standpoint of a partialist account that rests upon an account of relational responsibility, the question of the legacy of colonialism looks quite different. This is because, following Reader's analysis, the fact of relationship, the mutual constitutive effects of past colonial relationships, continues to create responsibilities. Relational responsibility begins where the 'reductio' of Ypi *et al.* ends. Here, then, is the final argument about why a relational responsibility approach is preferable. It is a better approach because it allows us to see a different and more serious set of harms, which grow out of power differentials in relationships of responsibility.

Relationships are often asymmetric. Even though relationships are constitutive, in some way, for all of the parties in the relationship, there is no reason to think that those relationships are equally meaningful, important, or central to the lives of each of the parties. Indeed, even in mutually beneficial relationships such as friendships (to say nothing of relationships of caring dependence), it is likely that one person is more needful in that relationship than others.

Several serious moral harms appear from this vantage point. One is the problem of dependency and the moral danger to the weaker party (or parties) in relationships of dependency (cf. Kittay 1999).[8] People who are weaker and in need of care are often at the mercy of those caring for them.

Another serious moral harm is the harm of abandonment. Leaving or breaking a relationship, especially by the powerful party, often causes great harm to the other party or parties. Indeed, so great is this harm that its seriousness is assumed and not thoroughly explored in the philosophical literature. Abandonment is often treated as an issue in professional ethics, that is, professionals should not abandon their charges (Panter-Brick 2000; Pellegrino 1995; Younggren & Gottlieb 2008). In the past, philosophers have described plant closings as morally harmful because they amount to a kind of abandonment (Kavanagh & Johnson 1982). To state that 'abandonment' has occurred seems already to describe a moral harm. Carol Gilligan offers some insight here when she posits that oppression and abandonment are the two great fears in human life (1996). When colonial powers left their colonies, did they abandon them? If so, does that moral harm create a strong form of responsibility? I would argue, from a relational responsibility perspective, given the ways in which colonial relationships have shaped people's lives, that it does.

Even without resort to the empirical facts about the harm of abandonment in particular cases, though, a relational account of responsibility can posit abandonment as a serious moral harm. Unilaterally to end relationships that entail responsibility creates a moral harm *on its face*. If we take seriously Walker's claim that responsibility requires a negotiation among the parties in the relationship, then simply to abandon a relationship is to forestall any renegotiation of existing responsibilities. It is, in this way, a moral harm. Thus, the emphasis on relationship and its connection to responsibility opens a different way to frame and consider questions of moral harms and justice in international relations.

A final objection should be considered. I have argued that partialist relational responsibilities best allow people to explore what they owe to others elsewhere in the world. This claim requires a deep and wide knowledge of one's dealings with the world. One advantage of universalistic claims, then, might be their relative simplicity. With one claim, one covers everybody. What about the partial nature of these relational responsibilities? After all, how can we be certain that all of the needy people will find themselves in some relationship that produces responsibility for their well-being? If many such individuals exist, then might this approach now fail to mitigate the harmful sufferings of them?

I admit that this claim raises an empirical question of whether the world is still populated by many Hobbesian humans, living in isolation or in bands, in some sort of state of nature, who have no relationships to others, or to states, or to other cultural or religious institutions. But until this ideological claim becomes an empirical one, I do not see why or how it should be given more force than the

---

8. An important theory of international relations, *dependencia*, promoted prominently by scholars in Latin America, used this argument to point to the large burden that Europeans and Americans from the United States owed to Latin Americans (Duvall 1978). While it is beyond the scope of this essay, this argument shows why that view was important.

alternative assumption with which I begin: humans always find themselves in relationships that produce responsibilities, and unless something goes horribly wrong in a person's/group's life, they remain within those relationships or create new ones. Those relations create and embody responsibility. All of those responsibilities, in their specific and far-reaching complexities are the grounds of moral life.

Conclusion

Our moral frameworks serve as a guide for our moral concerns and actions. In this paper I have made what may seem a counter-intuitive argument: starting from a partialist account of moral life that relies upon our concrete responsibilities provides a better guide to our global moral duties than does starting from a universalistic perspective that presumes 'wide but shallow' (Held 2008) commitments to all others.

I have argued that, given the complex nature of relationships of responsibility and the demands they place on us, we need to begin from a much more robust review of our responsibilities, including our abandoned and neglected responsibilities, in order to assess our moral concerns and action. By this account, partialist claims can be clarified so that they do not reach the status of being reductio ad absurdum, but they may prove to be disturbingly demanding.

Citizens in the Global North have a quite broad set of relations with people in the rest of the world, an elaboration of which is beyond the scope of this essay, but to establish this point we need only briefly think about how Reader (2003) describes the grounds of relation: for example, presence (e.g. by traveling abroad and having workers from abroad in their home states), biology (e.g. transnational kin), history (e.g. legacies of colonialism). Such relations thus create responsibilities. There will always be conflicts among these responsibilities and the pulls of different relations. Perhaps this complexity will work in favor of trying to open people up to taking these relations and responsibilities seriously. People who are used to recognizing the complexity and tragedy of their conflicting moral responsibilities might be willing to entertain the claims of forgotten or abandoned responsibilities more seriously. Invoking the everyday complexity of moral life, rather than blaming people for their failure to be more moral, might be a better way to proceed in trying to persuade people to care more for those around the world.

Many people believe that an ethic of care cannot provide a sufficiently broad or robust moral justification for considering global questions. I have suggested here that an account of relational responsibility can help us to move forward by asking citizens to begin the hard work of assessing their values and relationships, that is, by asking what they care about, what they must care for, how they must give care and respond to care-giving practices. To recognize how fundamental are our relationships of care requires a thoroughgoing rethinking of political life. If and only if democratic citizens can (a) see themselves as part of the process by which their nation acted, and (b) recognize levels and layers of responsibility, will they become ready and able to assume their global moral responsibilities. Citizens will always feel the need to 'protect themselves a little bit' (Norgaard 2006), but the question of how demands are made of them will help reassure them that their own real needs will not be sacrificed to those of others.

Such an approach is not universalistic in its construction, but it turns out to be radical and far-reaching in its effect. In the end, if we hope for citizens to recognize their global responsibilities, weak but universal ties may not be as useful as strong but partial genuine connections. Making those partial connections of relational responsibility more visible will lead the way to a more just world.

References

Duvall, R. D. (1978) 'Dependence and Dependencia Theory: Notes toward Precision of Concept and Argument', *International Organization*, Vol. 32, no. 1, pp. 51–78.

Esquith, S. L. (2010) *The Political Responsibilities of Everyday Bystanders*, Penn State University Press, State College, PA.

Feinberg, J. (1980) *Rights, Justice and the Bounds of Liberty*, Princeton University Press, Princeton.

Friedman, M. (1991) 'The Practice of Partiality', *Ethics*, Vol. 101, no. 4, pp. 818–35.

Gilligan, C. (1996) 'The Centrality of Relationship in Human Development: A Puzzle, Some Evidence, and a Theory', in *Development and Vulnerability in Close Relationships*, eds G. G. Noam & K. W. Fischer, Lawrence Erlbaum Associates, Mahwah, NJ, pp. 237–61.

Gould, C. C. (2004) *Globalizing Democracy and Human Rights*, Cambridge University Press, New York.

Haskell, T. L. (1998) *Objectivity is Not Neutrality: Explanatory Schemes in History*, Johns Hopkins University Press, Baltimore.

Held, V. (2008) *How Terrorism is Wrong: Morality and Political Violence*, Oxford University Press, New York.

Jaggar, A. (2005) 'Western Feminism and Global Responsibility', in *Feminist Interventions in Ethics and Politics*, eds B. S. Andrew, *et al.*, Rowman & Littlefield, Lanham, MD, pp. 185–200.

Kavanagh, J. P. & Johnson, E. W. (1982) 'Ethical Issues in Plant Relocation [with Commentary]', *Business and Professional Ethics Journal*, Vol. 1, no. 2, pp. 21–37.

Kittay, E. F. (1999) 'Love's Labor: Essays on Women, Equality and Dependency', ed. L. Nicolson, Routledge, New York.

Koggel, C. M. (1998) *Perspectives on Equality: Constructing a Relational Theory*, Rowman & Littlefield, Lanham, MD.

Leib, E. J. (2006) 'Responsibility and Social/Political Choices about Choice; or, One Way to Be a True Non-Voluntarist', *Law and Philosophy*, Vol. 25, no. 4, pp. 453–88.

McKenzie, C. & Stoljar, N. (eds) (2000) *Relational Autonomy: Feminist Essays on Autonomy, Agency, and the Social Self*, Oxford University Press, New York.

Miller, D. (2004) 'Holding Nations Responsible', *Ethics*, Vol. 114, no. 2, pp. 240–68.

Norgaard, K. M. (2006) '"People Want to Protect Themselves a Little Bit": Emotions, Denial, and Social Movement Nonparticipation', *Sociological Inquiry*, Vol. 76, no. 3, pp. 372–96.

Panter-Brick, C. (2000) 'Nobody's Children? A Reconsideration of Child Abandonment', in *Abandoned Children*, eds C. Panter-Brick & M. T. Smith, Cambridge University Press, New York, pp. 1–26.

Pellegrino, E. D. (1995) 'Nonabandonment: An Old Obligation Revisited', *Annals of Internal Medicine*, Vol. 122, no. 5, pp. 377–8.

Pogge, T. (2008) *World Poverty and Human Rights: Cosmopolitan Responsibilities and Reforms*, 2nd edn, Polity, Malden, MA.

Reader, S. (2003) 'Distance, Relationship and Moral Obligation', *Monist*, Vol. 86, no. 3, pp. 367–81.

Robinson, F. (1999) *Globalizing Care: Ethics, Feminist Theory, and International Relations*, Westview Press, Boulder.

Scheffler, S. (1997) 'Relationships and Responsibilities', *Philosophy and Public Affairs*, Vol. 26, no. 3, pp. 189–209.

Scheffler, S. (2001) *Boundaries and Allegiances: Problems of Justice and Responsibility in Liberal Thought*, Oxford University Press, New York.

Singer, P. (2002) *One World: The Ethics of Globalization*, Yale University Press, New Haven.

Smiley, M. (1992) *Moral Responsibility and the Boundaries of Community: Power and Accountability from a Pragmatic Point of View*, University of Chicago Press, Chicago.

Turoldo, F. & Barilan, M. Y. (2008) 'The Concept of Responsibility: Three Stages in its Evolution within Bioethics', *Cambridge Quarterly of Healthcare Ethics*, Vol. 17, no. 1, pp. 114–23.

Walker, M. (2006) *Moral Repair: Reconstructing Moral Relations after Wrongdoing*, Cambridge University Press, New York.

Walker, M. (2007) *Moral Understandings: A Feminist Study in Ethics*, 2nd edn, Oxford University Press, New York.

Young, I. M. (2006) 'Responsibility and Global Justice: A Social Connection Model', *Social Philosophy and Policy*, Vol. 23, no. 1, pp. 102–30.

Younggren, J. N. & Gottlieb, M. C. (2008) 'Termination and Abandonment: History, Risk, and Risk Management', *Professional Psychology: Research and Practice*, Vol. 39, no. 5, pp. 498–504.

Ypi, L., Goodin, R. E. & Barry, C. (2009) 'Associative Duties, Global Justice, and the Colonies', *Philosophy and Public Affairs*, Vol. 37, no. 2, pp. 103–35.

Index